Hydroxy-Pyridones as Antifungal Agents
with Special Emphasis on Onychomycosis

Springer
*Berlin
Heidelberg
New York
Barcelona
Hong Kong
London
Milan
Paris
Singapore
Tokyo*

S. Shuster (Ed.)

Hydroxy-Pyridones as Antifungal Agents with Special Emphasis on Onychomycosis

With 37 Figures

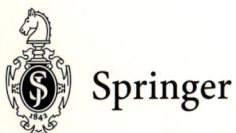
Springer

Sam Shuster, Emeritus Professor
University of Newcastle upon Tyne
Department of Dermatology
Framlington Place
Newcastle upon Tyne NE2 4HH
England

ISBN 3-540-65494-1 Springer-Verlag Berlin Heidelberg New York Tokyo

Library of Congress Cataloging-in-Publication Data
Hydroxy-pyridones as antifugal agents: with special emphasis on onychomycosis/Sam Shuster (ed.).
  p. cm.
  Includes bibliographical references.
  ISBN 3-540-65494-1 (softcover: alk. paper)
  1. Rilopirox. 2. Ciclopirox. 3. Onychomycosis–Chemotherapy.
I. Shuster, Sam.
RL 170.H93 1999   98-49275
615'.779–dc21   CIP

This work is subject to copyright. All rights are reserved, whether the whole or part of the material is concerned, specifically the rights of translation, reprinting, reuse of illustrations, recitation, broadcasting, reproduction on microfilm or in any other way, and storage in data banks. Duplication of this publication or parts thereof is permitted only under the provisions of the German Copyright Law of September 9, 1965, in its current version, and permission for use must always be obtained from Springer-Verlag. Violations are liable for prosecution under the German Copyright Law.

Springer-Verlag Berlin Heidelberg New York
a member of BertelsmannSpringer Science+Business Media GmbH

© Springer-Verlag Berlin Heidelberg 1999
Printed in Germany

The use of general descriptive names, registered names, trademarks, etc. in this publication does not imply, even in the absence of a specific statement, that such names are exempt from the relevant protective laws and regulations and therefore free for general use.

Product liability: The publishers cannot guarantee the accuracy of any information about the application of operative techniques and medications contained in this book. In every individual case the user must check such information by consulting the relevant literature.

Cover-Design: Design & Production GmbH, Heidelberg
Typesetting: K+V Fotosatz GmbH, Beerfelden

SPIN 10794562   18/3111 - 5 4 3 2 1 - Printed on acid-free paper

Preface

This book presents a series of papers on a special group of antifungal agents – the hydroxypyridones (e.g. Ciclopirox, Rilopirox, and Piroctone) given by international experts at conferences in Vancouver and Sydney.

The action of this group of agents is unique. Hydroxypyridones are not only active against all relevant fungi, but they are active against dermatophytes, yeasts, moulds as well as gram positive and gram negative bacteria. They have an inhibitory effect on the lipoxygenase and cyclo-oxygenase pathways and, in vitro, exhibit fungicidal and even sporicidal activity. Ciclopirox is particularly able to penetrate keratin.

These properties facilitate the treatment not only of tinea pedis caused by fungi but also of infections by gram negative bacteria. The special ability of Ciclopirox to penetrate keratin opens the door to an efficacious topical treatment for onychomycosis, with a transungual drug delivery system specially adapted to infections of the nail organ. The absence of drug interactions and systemic side effects of this formulation is an appreciable advantage over the newer systemic therapies for onychomycosis.

Papers are presented covering the mode of action, antimicrobial spectrum, pharmacological properties, penetration potential, clinical efficacy and the various indications for this group of drugs. They will enable the reader to assess the advantage and disadvantage of this new therapeutic modality.

We hope that the text will help to optimise the therapeutic approach to fungal infections of the skin in general and of onychomycosis in particular.

Contents

1 Hydroxy-Pyridones
  Outstanding Biological Properties
  A. MARKUS 1

2 Enzyme Histochemical Investigations of *Candida albicans*
  After Treatment with Rilopirox, a Novel Fungicidal
  Hydroxy-Pyridone
  H. K. REITZE, K.-A. SEITZ, D. R. DANNHORN, H. HÄNEL
  and M. BOHN 11

3 Can Ciclopirox Be Used as a Broad-Spectrum Anti-Infective
  Agent?
  W. SCHALLA, K. KRAEMER and R. POOTH 18

4 Studies of the Anti-Inflammatory Properties of Ciclopirox
  J. L. REES 33

5 Measurement of Ciclopirox Permeation Through Fingernail
  Models by Novel Spectroscopic Techniques
  T. M. BAYERL 36

6 Dermatomycosis: A Multifactorial Disease
  M. A. J. ALLEVATO 39

7 Efficacy of Topical Batrafen
  S. A. BUROVA 43

8 Ciclopirox Gel Treatment of Scalp Seborrhoeic Dermatitis
  B. B. ABRAMS, R. J. CHERILL, R. RAMASWAMY and H. I. KATZ 45

9 Seborrhoeic Dermatitis and Dandruff, and Its Treatment With
  Ciclopirox Shampoo
  S. SHUSTER 51

10 Epidemiology of Mycological Infections in Children –
   in South America
   F. M. GONZALEZ OTERO 56

11	Clinical Efficacy of Topical Ciclopirox Nail Lacquer: Double-Blind United States Studies on Onychomycosis R. Scher	62
12	Dose Regimen Studies with Ciclopirox Nail Lacquer G. Wozel	69
13	Open Studies of Ciclopirox Nail Lacquer in Onychomycosis – A Review S. Nolting	75
14	Influence of Onychomycosis on the Quality of Life A. Stary, S. Torma and P. G. Sator	81
15	Treatment of Onychomycosis: Pharmacoeconomic Aspects T. R. Einarson, P. I. Oh and N. Shear	91
16	The Safety Aspects of Systemic and Topical Antifungal Agents Used in the Management of Onychomycosis A. K. Gupta	96
17	Differential Diagnosis of Onychomycosis and Rationale for a Step-Therapy in Treating Nail Fungal Infection R. Baran	103

List of Contributors

Dr. Beatrice Abrams
Hoechst Marion Roussel Inc.
Clinical Research
Route 202–206
Bridgewater, NJ 08807-0800
USA

Dr. Miguel Angel J. Allevato
Jose M. Moreno 122-2° Piso Dto. 4
1424 Cap. Fed. Buenos Aires
Argentina

Dr. Robert Baran
Nail Disease Center
42, rue des Serbes
06400 Cannes
France

Dr. T.M. Bayerl
Universität Würzburg
Physikalisches Institut EP-5
Am Hubland
D-97074 Würzburg

Dr. S.A. Burova
Center of Deep Mycoses
Hospital N 81
Moscow
Russia

Dr. Thomas Einarson
19 Russell St.
Toronto, ON M5S 2S2
Canada

Dr. Aditya K. Gupta
490 Wonderland Road South, Suite 6
London, Ontario N6K 1L6
Canada

Dr. Astrid Markus
Central Pharmaceutical Research
Hoechst Marion Roussel
Deutschland GmbH
D-65926 Frankfurt

Dr. S. Nolting
Department of Dermatology
University Münster
Von-Esmarch-Strasse 56
D-48129 Münster

Dr. Francisco M. Gonzalez Otero
Department of Dermatology
School of Medicine
Caracas University Hospital
Venezuela

Professor Jonathan Rees
Department of Dermatology
University of Newcastle upon Tyne
Royal Victoria Infirmary
Newcastle upon Tyne NE1 4LP
England

Dr. H.K. Reitze
Philipps-University
Department of Zoology
Karl-von-Frisch-Strasse
D-35032 Marburg

Dr. Wolfgang Schalla
Dermatopharmacologic Laboratories
Rosastraße 9–13
D-79098 Freiburg

Dr. Richard Scher
25 Sutton Place South
New York, N.Y. 10022
USA

Sam Shuster, Emeritus Professor
Department of Dermatology
Framlington Place
University of Newcastle upon Tyne
NE2 4HH
England

Dr. Angelika Stary
Outpatients' Centre for Fungal
Infections and other Venero-
dermatological diseases
Franz Jonas-Platz 8-2-3
1210 Vienna
Austria

Dr. G. Wozel
Department of Dermatology
University Hospital
Carl Gustav Carus
Technical University Dresden
Fetscherstrasse 74
D-01307 Dresden

CHAPTER 1

Hydroxy-Pyridones

Outstanding Biological Properties

A. Markus

1.1
In Vitro

1.1.1
Biological Profile of Ciclopirox

Ciclopirox is a well-established antifungal, available in a number of topical formulations such as cream, solution, and powder. More recently, a nail lacquer for the topical treatment of onychomycosis has been introduced and marketed in many countries all over the world. In the following, I will first describe the antifungal potency of this drug and then explain why ciclopirox seems to be a perfect agent for the topical treatment of mycoses that develop in strongly hornified tissues.

Ciclopirox is a hydroxy-pyridone derivative that differs structurally and mechanistically from other known antimycotics. The antifungel activity is attributed to the hydroxy-pyridone group because the elimination of the hydroxy-substituent results in a compound that is completely inactive (Fig. 1.1).

1.1.2
Mode of Action

The mode of action has been carefully investigated and seems to be very complex, targeting a variety of metabolic processes in the fungal cell (Fig. 1.2). The basis of the main mechanism is the high affinity of ciclopirox for trivalent metal cations such as Fe^{3+}. The trapping of this essential enzymatic cofactor has an inhibitory effect on enzymes such as cytochromes, which are involved in mitochondrial electron transport processes in the course of energy production. In addition, the activity of catalase and peroxidase, which are responsible for the intracellular degradation of toxic peroxides, is strongly inhibited by the presence of the drug.

Earlier studies have shown that ciclopirox also impairs the fungal metabolism by affecting transport mechanisms located in the fungus cell membrane.

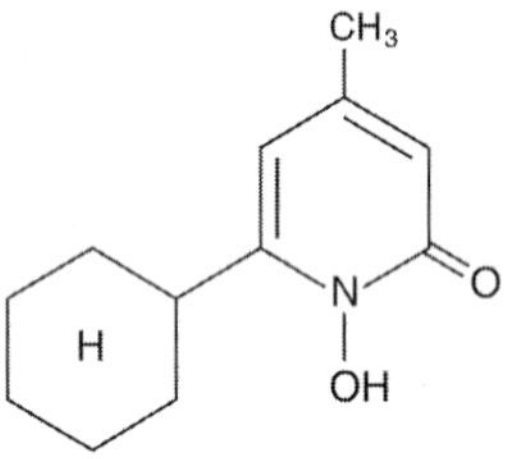

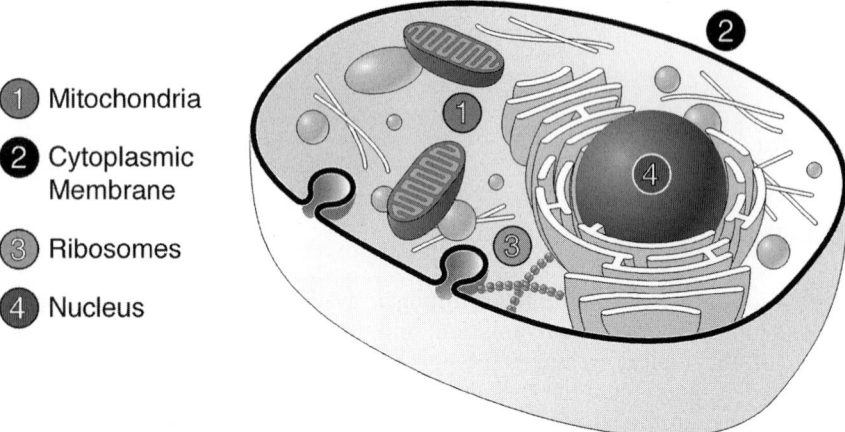

Fig. 1.1. Ciclopirox, the active substance of ciclopirox nail laquer

① Mitochondria
② Cytoplasmic Membrane
③ Ribosomes
④ Nucleus

Fig. 1.2. Ciclopirox: mode of action

A number of experiments have revealed that the uptake of nutrients into the internal pool is primarily affected. In growing cells, the intracellular depletion of essential amino acids and nucleotides secondarily contributes to the reduced synthesis of proteins or nucleic acids.

Owing to the complexity of the mechanism of action, the development of resistance against ciclopirox seems very unlikely.

1.1.3
Antifungal Spectrum

The antifungal activity of ciclopirox has been investigated by a number of different groups, all of which have found the compound to be a broad-spectrum antimycotic, active against many pathogenic dermatophytes, yeasts, and molds. Table 1.1 gives the minimum inhibitory concentrations taken from one representative study. The values indicated were determined by a macrodilution method.

Ciclopirox exhibits a well-balanced spectrum of activity, inhibiting all dermatophyte, yeast, and mold strains within a narrow concentration range. Dermatophytes, including important pathogens such as *Trichophyton, Microspor-*

Table 1.1. Antifungal spectrum of ciclopirox

Organisms (n)	Minimum inhibitory concentration (MIC) (µg/ml)						
	0.49	0.98	1.95	3.92	7.8	15.6	31.2
Trichophyton rubrum (37)	1	14	20	2			
Trichophyton mentagrophytes (29)		10	17	2			
Microsporum canis (20)	1	2	13	4			
Epidermophyton floccosum (5)		2	3				
Candida albicans (37)		21	11	5			
Candida tropicalis (12)		6	6				
Candida pseudotropicalis (9)			5	4			
Candida krusei (11)		2	8	1			
Candida parapsilosis (10)			5	5			
Other Candida spp. (6)		1	2	3			
Scopulariopsis brevicaulis (1)			1				
Aspergilli and other fungi (28)		1	9	10	3	5	
Scytalidium hyalinum (1)		1					
Fusarium solanae (1)							1

um, and *Epidermophyton spp.*, were inhibited at concentrations between 0.5 and 4 µg/ml. The same was true for all species of *Candida*, as well as for *Scopulariopsis brevicaulis*, which is also able to cause human nail infections. Most aspergilli and some other fungi were also sensitive between 1 and 4 µg/ml. The highest minimal inhibitory concentration (MIC) value was found in five of these strains and was 15.6 µg/ml.

1.1.4
Dose-Response Curve

There is a pronounced difference between the antifungal activity of hydroxy-pyridones and the azoles. In Fig. 1.3, the steepness of the growth response relationship was compared for ciclopirox and miconazole by using one strain of *Trichophyton mentagrophytes*. The results show that, under the experimental conditions used, the ciclopirox curve is much steeper than the curve obtained with miconazole. Although growth inhibition starts with ciclopirox at higher drug concentrations than with miconazole, a 100% growth inhibition is achieved with both drugs at similar concentration end points.

It is apparent that the activity of ciclopirox was hardly affected by the addition of protein. In contrast, the dose-response curve of miconazole became very flat when the medium was supplemented with 4% albumin, and very high miconazole concentrations were required to obtain complete growth inhibition.

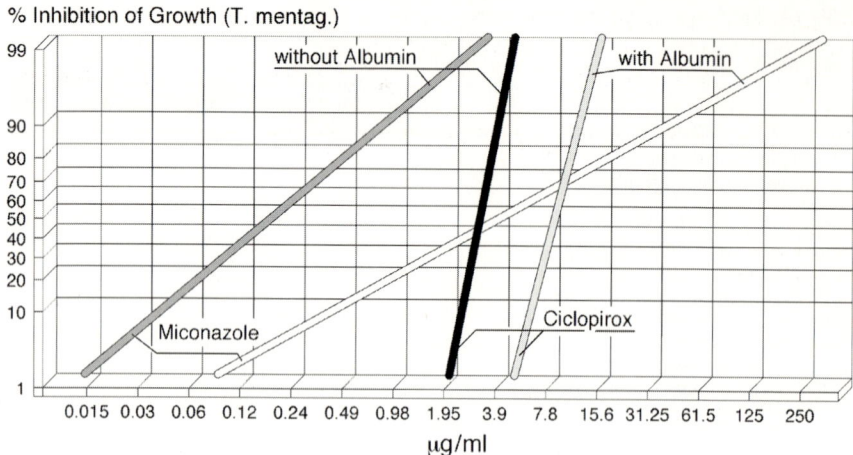

Fig. 1.3. Dose-response curve of ciclopirox and miconazole with and without 4% bovine serum albumin in agar medium

1.2
Fungicidal Activity

1.2.1
Proliferating Conditions

An important characteristic of the hydroxy-pyridones, which also distinguishes this class from that of the azoles, is their certain fungicidal potency, even against non-growing cells. This property is illustrated by the fact that fungal nail infection develops under conditions that do not promote optimal growth for the pathogen (Fig. 1.4).

A number of years ago, a publication reported that ciclopirox is able to kill *T. mentagrophytes* if the fungus is incubated in a complex medium in the presence of the drug. It was observed that the extent of fungicidal potency was dependent on both compound concentration and time. After 1 day of exposure, a 90% killing rate was achieved with 125 µg/ml ciclopirox. After 8 days of incubation in the presence of the drug, the viability of the pathogen was reduced by more than 99% at concentrations equal to the MIC.

1.2.2
Non-proliferating Conditions

Recent experiments have shown that the compound is also fungicidal against *T. mentagrophytes* when the experimental conditions do not promote fungal growth, e.g., when the incubation medium is buffer or water (Fig. 1.5).

We found that after 1 day of exposure more than 90% of the inoculated microconidia were killed in the presence of 640 µg/ml ciclopirox. A prolongation of the incubation time to 6 days reduced the concentration required to kill more than 90% of microconidia to 40 µg/ml.

Although these concentrations are generally higher than those found under optimal growth conditions, it was confirmed that there is indeed a correlation between the sporicidal effect and the incubation time.

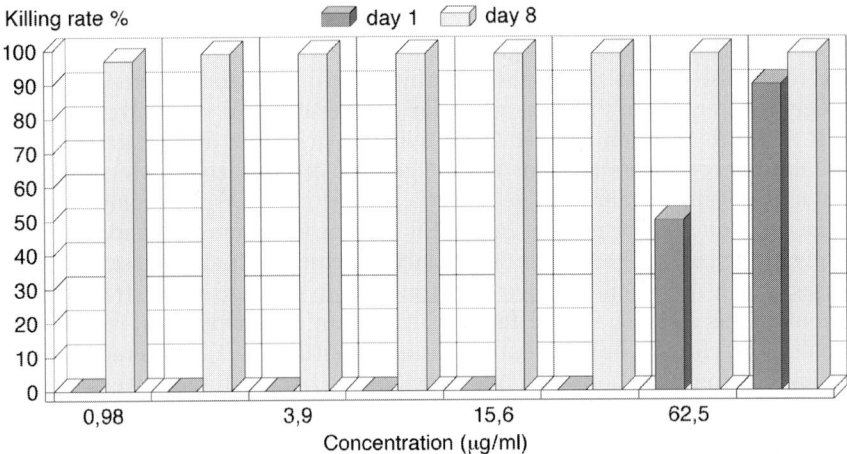

Fig. 1.4. Fungicidal activity of ciclopirox (proliferating conditions)

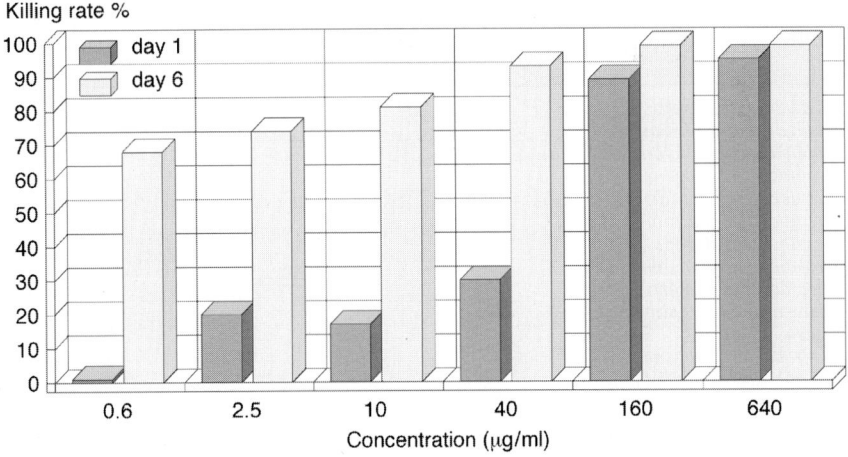

Fig. 1.5. Fungicidal activity of ciclopirox (non-proliferating conditions)

1.2.3
Antibacterial Activity

Under certain conditions, dermatomycoses might be complicated by secondary bacterial infections. Therefore, the antibacterial potency of ciclopirox was tested against a number of gram-positive and gram-negative aerobic bacteria, which are of importance with respect to superficial skin infections.

As can be seen from Table 1.2, ciclopirox is uniformly active against all strains, at concentrations ranging from 32 to 128 µg/ml. As expected, the spectrum also covers gram-positive strains with proven resistance against widely used antibiotics such as methicillin, ofloxacin, and vancomycin.

It is worth mentioning that the activity of ciclopirox against gram-negative strains represents a major advantage over certain azoles, which at best are active against gram-positive bacteria. In particular, *Pseudomonas aeruginosa* and *Proteus spp.* play an important part in the course of macerated interdigital mycoses. These bacteria produce enzymes such as elastase and proteases, which may facilitate their penetration into the macerated stratum corneum and, as a result, favor a further invasion by dermatophytes, yeasts, and molds. Therefore, a broad-spectrum antimicrobial, which, at therapeutically achievable concentrations, inhibits fungi as well as gram-negative bacteria, should be given preference for the treatment of mycoses that might be complicated by secondary gram-negative infections.

Table 1.2. Antibacterial spectrum of ciclopirox

Organisms (n)	MIC (µg/ml)					
	16	32	64	128	256	512
Gram-positive strains						
Staphylococcus aureus[a] (55)			47	8		
Staphylococcus epidermidis[a] (26)			6	20		
Streptococcus pyogenes (20)			20			
Streptococcus faecalis (3)			1	2		
Streptococcus faecium[a] (2)		1		1		
Streptococcus durans (10)			4	6		
Streptococcus equisimilis (1)				1		
Streptococcus agalactiae (9)				9		
Gram-negative strains						
Proteus vulgaris (3)		1	2			
Enterobacter aerogenes (1)				1		
Enterobacter cloacae (1)				1		
Escherichia coli (3)			3			
Klebsiella pneumoniae (2)			1	1		
Pseudomonas aeruginosa (5)				5		

[a] Including strains resistant to methicillin, ofloxacin, or vancomycin

1.2.4
Activity Against *Propionibacterium acnes*

As can be seen from Table 1.3, the antibacterial spectrum of ciclopirox also includes certain anaerobic bacteria such as *Propionibacterium acnes*. In an experiment using four strains of *P. acnes*, the antibacterial acitivities of ciclopirox and rilopirox were compared with those of erythromycin, gentamycin, and tetracyclin. It was found that all strains were uniformly inhibited by 32 µg/ml ciclopirox and 128 µg/ml rilopirox. Although the in vitro activity of ciclopirox is lower than that of the others, it seems, nevertheless, worthwhile to examine the therapeutic usefulness of ciclopirox in this indication, as the compound exhibits an excellent penetration behavior and certain anti-inflammatory properties, which might further support the therapeutic effect.

1.3
Penetration

Long-term experience has shown, that the penetration behavior of antifungal formulations can be reliably tested in vitro by using the excised skin of animals such as pigs or by using artificial cow horn slices. In the following, the figures (Figs. 1.6–1.8) are divided into two parts, illustrating the experimental method schematically on the *left*, and the respective result on the right. The results were gained from experiments conducted at Hoechst.

1.3.1
Penetration: Pigskin Model

In the first experiment, we used three pieces of skin from the backs of pigs that had been treated on the epidermis either with ciclopirox nail lacquer or with the drug-free vehicle, or that remained untreated and served as a growth control (Fig. 1.6).

After 2-min exposure, the lacquers were removed with adhesive tape. Subsequently, the epidermis of each skin piece was cut into three sections, and

Table 1.3. Antibacterial acitivity of ciclopirox against anaerobes

Organism	Minimum inhibitory concentration MIC (µg/ml)				
	Ciclopirox olamine	Rilopirox	Erythro-mycin	Genta-micin	Tetra-cycline
Propionibacterium acnes 6919	32	128	0.062	8	0.25
P. acnes 6922	32	128	0.062	8	0.25
P. acnes 15549	32	128	0.062	8	0.25
P. acnes DSM 20458	32	64	0.031	1	0.125

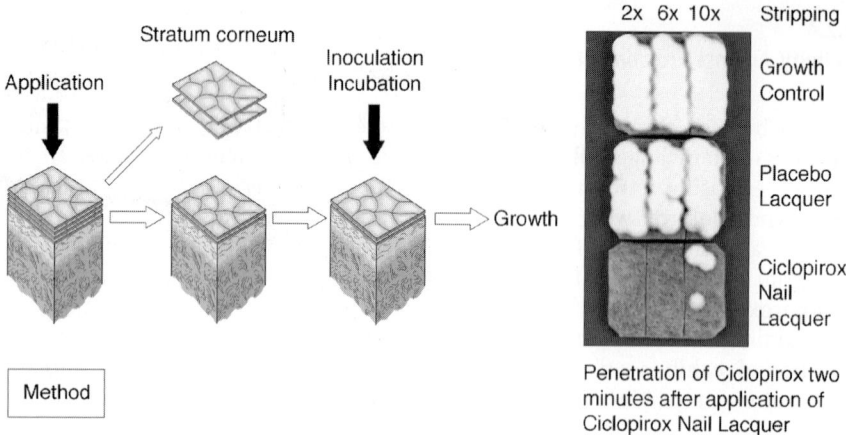

Fig. 1.6. Penetration of ciclopirox through the stratum corneum of skin (pigskin)

the stratum corneum was stripped using adhesive tape. The first section was stripped twice, the second area 6 times, and the third area 10 times. In order to investigate the penetration and antifungal potency of ciclopirox in the various layers of the stratum corneum, all areas were uniformly inoculated with *T. mentagrophytes*. After 7 days of incubation at 28°C, fungal growth occurred on all areas of the untreated skin as well as on the skin piece that had been treated with the placebo lacquer.

The skin piece that had been treated with ciclopirox nail lacquer was free of fungal growth on the first two segments and exhibited only a few colonies on the area that had been stripped 10 times.

This experiment indicates that antifungal drug concentrations are liberated from the lacquer formulations and rapidly penetrate into deeper layers of the stratum corneum, where they display full antimycotic activity.

1.3.2
Penetration: Cow Horn Model

Another experiment, using cow horn slices, was performed to demonstrate the penetration of ciclopirox even through highly keratinized tissue (Fig. 1.7). One slice was treated on the upper side with ciclopirox nail lacquer, a second slice remained untreated and served as a growth control. After the lacquer had been dried, the reverse sides of the slices were inoculated with *T. mentragrophytes*.

After a 10-day incubation at 28°C, uniform fungal growth was visible on the control slice. On the treated slice, a clear inhibition zone was visible, corresponding to the area where the ciclopirox lacquer had been applied to the reverse side.

This experiment again indicates that the lacquer promotes the penetration of ciclopirox through keratin.

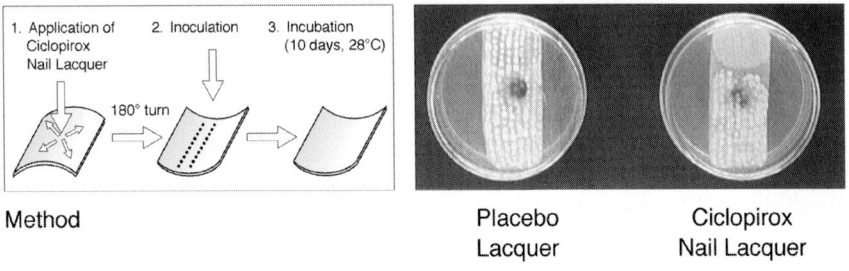

Fig. 1.7. Penetration of ciclopirox through keratin (cow horn)

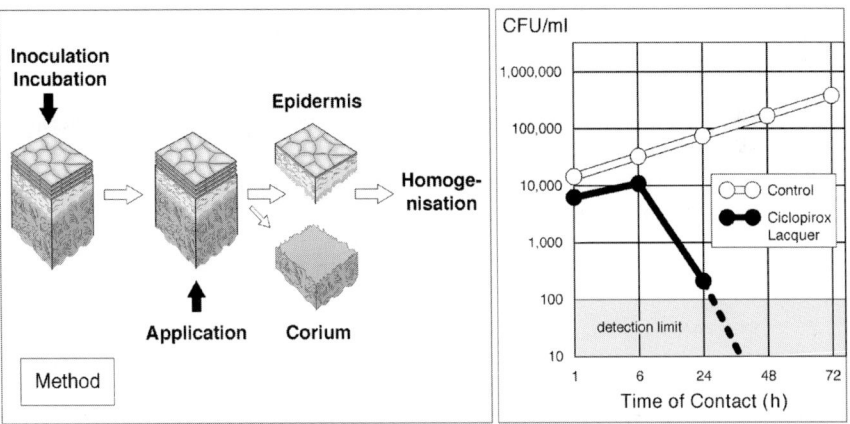

Fig. 1.8. Fungicidal activity of ciclopirox nail laquer against *Trichophyton mentagrophytes* at the site of infection (skin model)

1.3.3
Fungicidal Activity (Pigskin Model)

In a third penetration experiment, we wanted to show that the lacquer acts not only by growth inhibition, but is also fungicidal. Therefore, we investigated whether the lacquer formulation is able to reduce the number of viable fungal elements in the epidermis of infected skin (Fig. 1.8).

In a first step, *T. mentagrophytes* was allowed to grow on the epidermis of several skin pieces for a few days, before the nail lacquer was applied to the bottom of the skin. At certain time intervals, the epidermis, which contained the fungal elements, was separated from the cutis, and the viable cell counts were determined in epidermal homogenates, using a conventional agar-plating technique.

On the right, Fig. 1.8 shows that there was a clear correlation between the time the lacquer had been in contact with the infected skin and the decrease in viable counts in the epidermis. After a 24-h contact, the number of colony-forming units was reduced by more than 2 log steps in comparison with the respective non-treated control. After 48 and 72 h, no viable fungal elements could be detected, i.e., the number of viable fungal cells in the epidermis had been reduced to below the detection limit of the method.

1.4
Summary

- Ciclopirox exhibits a unique and complex mode of action, which mainly affects iron-dependent enzyme systems (e.g., cytochromes, catalase, peroxidase) and the cytoplasmic membrane (e.g., transport mechanisms).
- Ciclopirox is uniformly active against human pathogenic fungi with very steep dose-response curves. In addition, it is active against gram-positive and gram-negative bacteria including antibiotic-resistant strains.
- Ciclopirox has fungicidal and sporicidal activity in vitro.
- Ciclopirox demonstrates excellent penetration properties through keratin. Several in vitro experiments with nail lacquer applied to hornified tissues (skin, cow horn) confirmed drug liberation, penetration, and antifungal activity at the site of infection.

CHAPTER 2

Enzyme Histochemical Investigations of *Candida albicans* After Treatment with Rilopirox, a Novel Fungicidal Hydroxy-Pyridone

H. K. REITZE, K.-A. SEITZ, D. R. DANNHORN, H. HÄNEL and M. BOHN

2.1
Introduction

Rilopirox (HOE 351) is a hydroxy-pyridone compound with antimycotic properties. Hydroxy-pyridones are generally active against medically important dermatophytes, yeasts and moulds, and they exhibit a significant fungicidal potency even against non-proliferating fungal cells and spores.

Hydroxy-pyridone derivatives have a strong chelating potential, which seems to play an important role in their antifungal mode of action. Rilopirox inactivates metal ion-dependent fungal enzymes and proteins from *Saccharomyces cerevisiae*-like cytochromes of the respiratory chain as well as catalase (Kruse et al. 1991). These data are supported by observations that after treatment with rilopirox the intracellular concentration of the cytotoxic agent hydrogen peroxide is increased in *Candida albicans* (Laskin 1994).

2.2
Aim of the Study

On the basis of these results, indicating a severe impairment of energy metabolism and hydrogen peroxide degradation of the fungus, we performed two series of studies at the ultrahistochemical level.

In a first study, we investigated the influence of rilopirox on the two metal ion-dependent enzymes, catalase and peroxidase, as well as on the non-enzymatic protein cytochrome c. In a second study, we evaluated the effect of rilopirox on acid phosphatase, an unspecific hydrolytic enzyme complex that is involved in degradative processes.

2.3
Materials and Methods

The test organism *C. albicans*, strain 200/175 (Hoechst), was suspended in casein hydrolysate-dextrose liquid medium. After a preincubation period of

24 h, rilopirox was added to final drug concentrations of 1, 10 and 20 µg/ml, respectively. One, 6 and 24 h after inoculation, the yeast cells were harvested by centrifugation and prepared for cytochemical investigations.

For the detection of enzyme activity, the samples were generally fixed with glutaraldehyde, using different concentrations and pH values, depending on the subsequent enzyme analysis. The various enzyme activities were detected using modified standard techniques: catalase (Novikoff and Goldfisher 1969), peroxidase (Graham and Karnovsky 1966), cytochrome c (Karnovsky and Rice 1969), and acid phosphatase (Barka and Anderson 1962).

Preparation of the samples for ultrastructural analysis was carried out with specific methods developed in our own laboratory (Mothes-Wagner et al. 1984). Normally, ultrathin sections were poststained with potassium permanganate and lead citrate (Reynolds 1963) in order to visualize membrane structures. As a control, some sections of each series remained unstained.

2.4
Results

2.4.1
Catalase and Peroxidase

After incubation in a specific medium for the detection of catalase activity, the reaction product in the control cells could be found not only in the peroxisome-like bodies but also in the mitochondria. The electron opaque precipitate is clearly visible in the matrix of the peroxisome-like bodies as well as on the membrane system of the mitochondria in both poststained and unstained sections (Fig. 2.1a).

The staining reaction inside the peroxisome-like bodies is probably owing to a true catalase activity, since no precipitation is detectable in these organelles in sections treated with the specific catalase inhibitor, aminotriazole. The simultaneous oxidation of diaminobenzidine by mitochondria, however, insensitive to aminotriazole, is interpreted as indicative for the presence of a mitochondrial peroxidase (Threadgold and Read 1968; Hoffmann et al. 1970).

With regard to the peroxisome-like bodies, and independent of the concentrations investigated, no remarkable reduction in the intensity of the reaction product is visible after exposure to rilopirox for up to 6 h. Inside the mitochondria, however, first structural changes with a reduced amount of precipitate are already seen after treatment with rilopirox for 1 h (Fig. 2.1b,c). Therefore, it seems very likely that the compound primarily affects the activity of mitochondrial peroxidase.

Incubation with rilopirox for 24 h resulted in the degeneration and often total lysis of most of the evaluated yeast cells, independent of the actual concentration. In these highly necrotic cells, the reaction product is nearly absent and restricted only to a few membrane fractions of the mitochondria (Fig. 2.1d).

In summary, the catalase activity in peroxisome-like bodies was only inhibited in yeast cells treated for 24 h, independent of the concentrations of

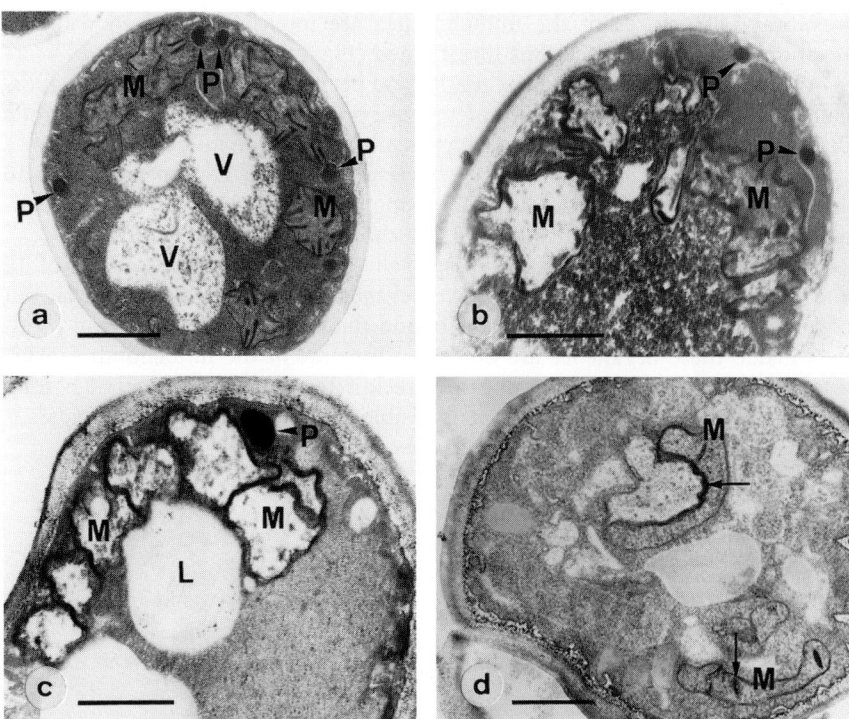

Fig 2.1 a–d. Localization of catalase and peroxidase activity after exposure to rilopirox. **a** Poststained control section showing reaction products on the cristae and the limiting membranes of the mitochondria (*M*) as well as on the small peroxisome-like bodies (*P*). (*N*, nucleus; *V*, vacuolar system) (*bar*=1 µm). **b** 20 µg/ml rilopirox for 1 h, poststained section. Enlarged and deformed mitochondria (*M*) exhibiting a reduced amount of reaction product on fractionated cristae and surrounding membranes. Small peroxisome-like bodies (*arrowsheads*) located at the cell periphery are still reactive (*bar*=1 µm). **c** 20 µg/ml rilopirox for 6 h, poststained section. Accumulation of strongly damaged mitochondria (*M*) near the cell periphery exhibiting reaction product only on limiting membranes. The cristae and the matrix of the organelles are disintegrated. However, a small peroxisome-like body (*P*) is still labelled, indicating enzyme reaction. (*L*, lipid) (*bar*=1 µm). **d** 1 µg/ml rilopirox for 24 h, poststained section. Cellular equipment of the yeast cell extremely damaged. Deformed mitochondria (*M*) without cristae. The reaction product is restricted to certain parts of the surrounding membranes (*arrows*) (*bar*=1 µm)

rilopirox investigated. A reduced amount of the reaction product in mitochondria, indicating peroxidase activity, was already detectable after 6 h of treatment with all concentrations of rilopirox used.

2.4.2
Cytochrome *c*

The localization of the diaminobenzidine reaction product, indicating the presence of cytochrome *c*, is restricted to the mitochondrial cristae and the limiting membranes in both poststained and unstained control sections. The membrane structures of the mitochondria are intensively labelled with the reaction product in all sections investigated (Fig. 2.2a).

After treatment with rilopirox for 1 h, no peculiar alterations of the cell organelles occur, but the intensity of the reaction product seems to be slightly diminished, especially on the limiting membranes of the mitochondria.

After an incubation time of 6 h, however, the drug concentrations of 10 and 20 µg/ml, respectively, cause increasing cellular damage, and the precipitate is located only sporadically on a few shortened cristae (Fig. 2.2b,c).

Exposure to rilopirox for 24 h, especially with drug concentrations of 10 and 20 µg/ml, results in a progressive degeneration of the mitochondria, but considerable variations in the intensity and the location of the reaction products inside these organelles are obvious. One part of the mitochondria exhibits an extremely reduced amount of precipitate, whereas in others a strong deposition of the reaction product is visible inside the matrix but not associated with the mitochondrial membranes (Fig. 2.2d).

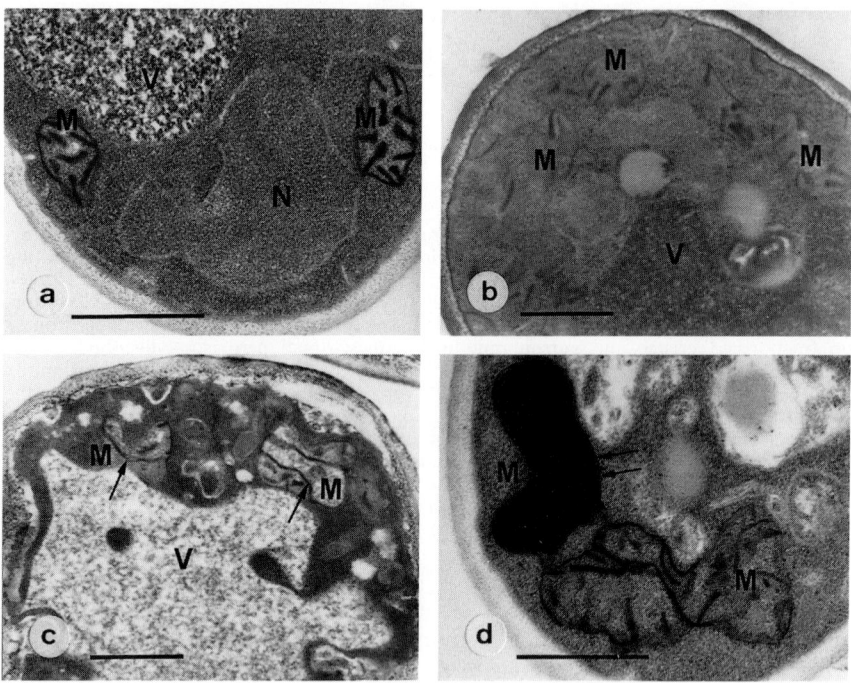

Fig. 2.2a–d. Localization of cytochrome *c* after exposure to rilopirox. **a** Mitochondria (*M*) of the poststained control cell show strong depositions of the precipitate. Other organelles are not labelled. (*V*, vacuolar system; *N*, nucleus) (*bar*=1 µm). **b** 10 µg/ml rilopirox for 6 h, poststained section. The electron opaque reaction product can be sporadically detected on the mitochondrial cristae (*M*). (*V*, vacuolar system) (*bar*=1 µm). **c** 20 µg/ml rilopirox for 6 h, poststained section. Yeast cell exhibiting an extended vacuolar system (*V*). The precipitate is present on a few cristae (*arrows*) of the rather damaged mitochondria (*M*) (*bar*=1 µm). **d** 20 µg/ml rilopirox for 24 h, poststained section. The mitochondria (*M*) are intensively labelled for cytochrome *c*. An increasing amount of the reaction product is additionally found inside the matrix of these organelles (*arrows*) (*bar*=1 µm)

Taken together, 6 h of treatment with 10 and 20 µg/ml rilopirox resulted in increased cellular damage, and the precipitate demonstrating cytochrome c was located only in a few shortened mitochondrial christae.

The effects of rilopirox were most prominent after 24 h of treatment. Some mitochondria exhibited an extremely reduced amount of precipitate associated with the membranes, whereas in others a strong deposition of the precipitate was visible in the mitochondrial matrix.

2.4.3
Acid Phosphatase

In untreated control cells, the lead phosphate precipitate that indicates acid phosphatase activity is observed exclusively at the outer surface of the cell wall. The cell wall itself, as well as the interior of the cell, are devoid of the reaction product (Fig. 2.3a). Control samples incubated in medium lacking the substrate are nearly free of precipitation.

Exposure to 1 µg/ml rilopirox for 1 h results in only minimal differences in the intensity and distribution of the reaction product. The exposure to 20 µg/ml rilopirox for 1 h results in a separation of the cell membrane from the cell wall, and a prominent amount of reaction product is additionally located inside the generating space. Simultaneously, the reaction product at the outer surface of the cells is diminished (Fig. 2.3b).

After treatment of *C. albicans* with 20 µg/ml rilopirox for 6 h, a markedly reduced amount of the reaction product is seen at the outer surface of the cell wall. On the other hand, the deposition of the reaction products between the cell wall and the plasma membrane as well as inside the vacuolar system is strongly increased (Fig. 2.3c). The same reaction pattern can be seen in sections of yeast cells treated with the minimal drug concentration of 1 µg/ml rilopirox for 24 h.

Treatment with 10 µg/ml for 24 h results in formation of a continuous space between the cell wall and the plasma membrane, which is entirely filled with the reaction product. Beyond that, the precipitate forms aggregates inside the vacuolar system.

After exposure to 20 µg/ml, nearly all cells investigated are highly necrotic after an incubation period of 24 h. However, in spite of the enhanced degradation of the yeast cells, the remaining membrane fractions of the vacuolar system are still intensively stained for acid phosphatase activity (Fig. 2.3d).

In summary, 1 h of treatment with 20 µg/ml rilopirox resulted in a decrease in enzyme activity at the surface of the cell wall and a concomitant increase in activity between the cell wall and the cell membrane.

In addition to the effects visible after 1 h of treatment, 20 µg/ml rilopirox achieved a marked increase in enzyme activity inside the vacuolar system after a 6-h incubation period.

Exposure to 20 µg/ml for 24 h resulted in highly necrotic cells. In spite of this, an intensive staining of enzyme activity is still detectable, associated with the membrane fractions of the yeast cells.

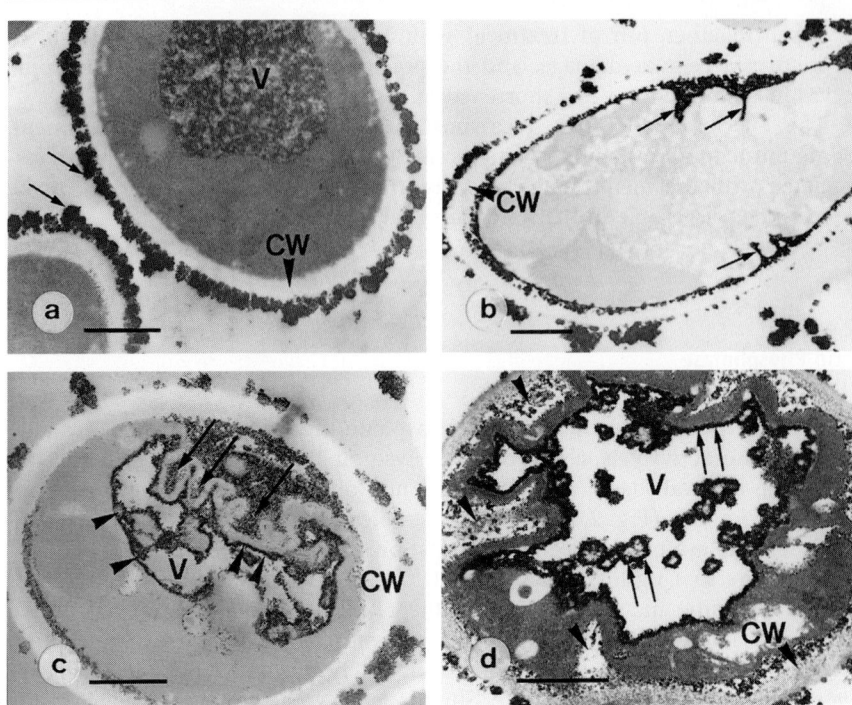

Fig. 2.3 a–d. Localization of acid phosphatase activity after exposure to rilopirox. **a** Poststained control section. The reaction product is exclusively located outside the yeast cells (*arrows*), forming a continuous electron dense coat on the surface of the cell wall (*CW*). (*V*, vacuolar system) (*bar*=1 μm). **b** 20 μg/ml rilopirox for 1 h. The unstained section shows a reduced amount of precipitate on the outer cell surface. Granulated precipitate appears between the cell wall (*CW*) and the plasmalemma, forming elongated invaginations in some regions (*arrows*) (*bar*=1 μm). **c** 20 μg/ml rilopirox for 6 h, unstained section. The precipitate is located in the large space between the cell wall (*CW*) and the plasmalemma, forming partial deep invaginations into the cytoplasm (*arrows*). The adjacent vacuolar system (*V*) exhibits precipitate on the bordering membrane (*arrowheads*). Only a few aggregates of reaction product are still visible at the cell surface (*bar*=1 μm). **d** 20 μg/ml rilopirox for 24 h, poststained section. A strong deposition of reaction product is seen on the limiting membrane of the vacuolar system (*V*) and on the surface of vesicles (*arrows*) located in the vacuolar lumen. The precipitate between the cell wall (*CW*) and the plasmalemma is apparently reduced (*arrowheads*) (*bar*=1 μm)

2.5
Conclusions

In conclusion, the pattern of damage identified in *C. albicans* after exposure to rilopirox indicates different targets of the hydroxy-pyridone compound on the ultrastructural and enzyme histochemical level:

1. The impairment of catalase activity in peroxisome-like bodies followed by an intracellular increase in hydrogen peroxide concentration may be finally involved in the autolysis of the yeast cells.

2. The inhibition of mitochondrial peroxidase activity suggests an impairment of the respiratory chain reactions, resulting in an insufficient energy supply to the yeast cells.
3. At least two different effects on the small carrier protein cytochrome c of the respiratory chain are suggested: The cytochrome c function is reduced and/or the association of cytochrome c to mitochondrial membranes is impaired.
4. The enhancement of phosphatase activity inside the vacuole and between the cell membrane and the cell wall supports the idea that this is part of a non-specific defense mechanism concerning elimination and digestion of lytic material.
5. It is suggested that the secretory pathway of acid phosphatases to the outer surface of the cell wall is disturbed by rilopirox, followed by an intracellular activation of hydrolase precursors ("sleeping enzymes") that may finally result in a complete cellular breakdown.

References

Barka T, Anderson PJ (1962) Histochemical methods for acid phosphatase using hexazonium pararosanilin as coupler. J Histochem Cytochem 10:741

Graham RC, Karnovsky MJ (1966) The early stages of absorption of injected horseradish peroxidase in the proximal tubules of mouse kidney. Ultrastructural cytochemistry by a new technique. J Histochem Cytochem 14:291

Hoffmann H-P, Szabo A, Avers CJ (1970) Cytochemical localization of catalase activity in yeast peroxisomes. J Bacteriol 104:581–584

Karnovsky MJ, Rice DF (1969) Exogenous cytochrome c as an ultrastructural tracer. J Histochem Cytochem 17:751

Kruse R, Hengstenberg W, Hänel H, Raether W (1991) Studies for the elucidation of the mode of action of the antimycotic hydroxypyridone compound rilopirox. Pharmacology 43:247–255

Laskin JD (1994) Peroxide production by human keratinocytes and Candida albicans in response to the antifungal agents rilopirox and cyclopirox. Report August 1994

Mothes-Wagner U, Wagner G, Reitze HK, Seitz K-A (1984) A standardized technique for the in toto epoxy resin embedding and precipitate-free staining of small specimens covered by strong protective outer surface. J Microsc 134: 307–313

Novikoff AB, Goldfischer S (1969) Visualization of peroxisomes (microbodies) and mitochondria with diaminobenzidine. J Histochem Cytochem 17:675–685

Reynolds ES (1963) The use of lead citrate at high pH as an electron opaque stain in electron microscopy. J Cell Biol 17:208–212

Threadgold LT, Read CP (1968) Electron microscopy of Fasciola hepatica. V. Peroxidase localization. Exp Parasitol 23:221

CHAPTER 3

Can Ciclopirox Be Used as a Broad-Spectrum Anti-Infective Agent?

W. SCHALLA, K. KRAEMER and R. POOTH

3.1
Introduction

Most bacterial habitants of the skin surface do not induce clinical symptoms and are therefore regarded as part of the normal flora. However, although they may be harmless for a healthy host, whether as transients or as part of the resident skin and mucosal flora, a pathological state develops if these facultatively pathogenic bacteria enter the body, particularly in severely ill patients with reduced defense mechanisms or in autoimmune responses. The former explains so-called hospital infections; the latter depends on the entry site of the bacteria and the strain subtype [reviews in 1–6].

Staphylococcus aureus is found in 20%–40% of healthy individuals on the nasal mucosa, and on the skin of the perineal and/or the axillary region in up to 60% of the hospital staff. The latter group of bacterial carriers is important as a source of hospital infections, particularly since these carriers often carry multiresistant strains, in contrast to the normal population.

The *mode of entry* is crucial, and this is underlined by the fact that throat infections rather than skin infections by *Streptococcus pyogenes* induce rheumatic diseases. The horny layer protects very efficiently against infections of *Staphylococcus aureus* and *Streptococcus pyogenes*, since no infections could be initiated by inoculating even high numbers of microorganisms (up to 10^7 organisms) under occlusion. The number of *Streptococcus pyogenes* on the normal skin surface spontaneously dropped drastically within 24 h, be it on lipid-poor or lipid-rich areas. A breach in the integrity of the skin appears to be an absolute requirement for infection. No difference exists between very superficial skin damage by non-bleeding scratching and deeper scarification leading to pin-point bleeding. Such superficial wounds do not develop into ecthyma, regional lymphadenitis and fever. This only occurs if large numbers of *Streptococcus pyogenes* (10^7 organisms) are implanted into the *deep* dermis (although this was done in just one subject [7]), or if smaller amounts are transported into the deep dermis in the presence of other foreign substances that add insult to the original injury such as insect bites or surgical sutures [7, 11].

Different strains of the same species may behave differently. *Age* also seems to play a major role. Postinfection nephritis occurs principally in preschool children and exempts adults. The host develops an immunity that lasts for some years and seems to be related to M protein [1].

Infections of superficial skin wounds by *Staphylococcus aureus* or *Streptococcus pyogenes* are followed by very localized pyodermas such as impetigo and folliculitis, and some strains of *Streptococcus pyogenes* can cause erysipelas. Although the different types of pyoderma are self-limiting in terms of spreading and duration of the infection, it is necessary to treat these skin diseases.

Ciclopirox inhibits in vitro growth of fungi, mycoplasms, *Trichomonas* species, and gram-positive and a number of gram-negative bacteria, and is therefore a good candidate as a broad-spectrum anti-infective agent. In skin infections, drug availability may, however, be diminished by pus and crust formation, inactivation by binding and metabolization, etc.

To study the influence of most of the in vivo factors (Table 3.1) on the antibacterial activity, we used two types of artificially induced superficial pyodermas, since naturally occurring pyodermas are quite variable in their nature, evolution, and time course and would require many patients to prove the expected efficacy. In addition, the virulence of naturally occurring strains is not known. The risk of secondary complications in patients seems thereby unreasonably high during this investigational period in view of the fact that experimentally induced pyodermas use strains with known virulence and need only a few healthy volunteers [7]. The inclusion of a vehicle control (placebo), as demanded by several health authorities, is also more conveniently performed in healthy subjects than in patients.

This established standardized human pyoderma model uses laboratory strains and an epicutaneous route of infection to give well-characterized localized pyodermic reactions and a close surveillance of the antimicrobial treatment. The effects can be compared in an intraindividual test design, with a known effective topical antibiotic agent as positive control. Leyden et al. [11] demonstrated in a previous study with a 2% mupirocin ointment (Bactroban) that this test design allows reliable measurements of topical antibiotic efficacy in a few healthy volunteers.

Table 3.1. In vivo factors

Penetration barriers	• Horny layer • Fibrin wall • Crusts • Fibrosis/sclerosis
Inflammation	• Vasodilation • Edema/bullae • Inflammatory cells • Pus/pustules
Mixed infections	• Athlete's foot • *Staphylococcus aureus* + *Candida albicans*

3.2
Methods

3.2.1
Inoculation

Artificial pyodermas were induced in 24 healthy Caucasian subjects with a mean age of 34 years (range 19–61) by the procedures described by Leyden [11], which consist in the following steps:
- Damage of skin on the forearms
- Inoculation with *Staphylococcus aureus/Streptococcus pyogenes* [10^7 germs/ 10 µl applied]
- Incubation for 24 h
- Treatment 3 times a day for 5 days (days 0–5)
- Clinical scoring (days 0–5, day 7, day 21)
- Quantitative culture count (day 1, day 5, day 7)

The breach in the horny layer barrier was done by scarification in the case of *Streptococcus pyogenes* and by using the base of ammonium hydroxide blisters [8] after a rest period of 24 h under occlusion in the case of *Staphylococcus aureus*.

Streptococcus pyogenes: four scratched test fields on the forearm were inoculated by a laboratory strain for 24 h leading to papulopustules without major crusts. *Staphylococcus aureus:* NH_4OH blisters were raised on four test sites on the other forearm, the blister roof removed, and after a 24-h rest period the ground inoculated for 24 h, resulting mainly in pus and crust formation.

The in vivo behavior of the strains used was known from previous experiments and the sensitivity to the two active drugs was tested using standard in vitro procedures. Stock cultures of the strains were subcultured at least twice before use to regain virulence, as proposed by Leyden et al. [7].

3.2.2
Treatment

After the inoculation period, one test site of either pyoderma type served as untreated control. Three others were treated thrice daily for 5 days in a double-blind, randomized manner by 1% ciclopirox cream (Batrafen), the cream base, and 2% mupirocin ointment (Turixin), respectively.

Glucocorticoids, antimycotics, antibiotics, anti-infectives, antimetabolites, immunostimulants, or immunosuppressives had not to be given from 3 weeks prior to the study up to the end – neither topical on the arms nor systemically.

3.2.3
Efficacy Criteria

The lesions were scored from 0 (none/not present) to 4 (most severe) for erythema, papulopustules, pus formation, edema/infiltration, and crusts/scaling at the start of treatment (day 0), once daily during and at the end of treatment (days 1–5), and twice at follow-up (days 7 and 21).

For counting, bacteria were sampled from the infected sites by the detergent scrub technique [9] at 24 h after the start, at the end of treatment, and 2 days thereafter. Then followed serial dilutions; plating on sheep's blood, mannitol, and colistin-nalidixin agar, respectively; incubation at 37°C for 24 h; and finally counting the number of colony-forming units (CFU).

3.2.4
Safety Variables

Local irritation reactions could represent contact allergies or non-specific overreactions to the organism, or to the study medication. They were recorded, as were the spreading of a pyoderma beyond an area measuring fivefold that of the initial area and other types of adverse events.

Hematology, blood biochemistry, clinical immunology (C-reactive protein, antistreptolysin, rheumatoid factor, antistreptodornase B, antihyaluronidase, antistaphylolysin), and urinalysis were done at precheck and at the end of the follow-up period in addition to regular checks for signs of infections in general and for those of the respiratory and urinary tract in particular.

3.2.5
Statistics

The results in the literature [11] indicate that the intraindividual differences of the logarithms of the microorganism counts have a standard deviation of approximately 0.4. Therefore, a two-sided one-sample t-test at level 0.05 for these intraindividual differences would detect a delta of 0.25 with a power of 0.86 using a sample size of 24 subjects. This corresponds to a ratio of 1.78 between treatments for the microorganism count itself (not the logarithm).

An α-adjustment owing to multiple-treatment effect comparisons was not necessary since the quantity of recovered bacteria after 24 h of treatment was taken as the primary end point, all other variables compared as secondary ones. The two types of infection were regarded as independent scientific investigations, and hence there was one treatment comparison of primary interest.

Treatment differences in the bacterial counts were tested by analysis of variance (ANOVA) after log-transformation using the 24-h-values (day 1) as the main criterion, and treatment and subject as fixed effect at the two-sided α-level of 5%. Additionally, two-sided 95% confidence intervals were calculated for the treatment contrast. The contrast mupirocin minus control was used to assess the sensitivity (responsiveness) of the pyoderma model, and the contrast vehicle minus control was used to test for a vehicle effect. The bacterial counts and the clinical scores at the end of treatment (day 5) were taken as secondary efficacy criteria.

The clinical scores at the end of treatment were analyzed without log-transformation by ANOVA for treatment differences. For the comparison of ciclopirox olamine cream and its vehicle, McNemar's test was used in addition with one-sided p values derived from the exact binomial distribution, since the assumption of a normal distribution for the symptom intensity scores is questionable. Measurements for the non-parametric analysis were classified as "ciclopirox cream better than vehicle," "no difference," or "ciclopirox cream worse than vehicle" for each subject.

3.2.6
Good Clinical Practice

The study was assessed positively by an independent Ethics Committee and carried out in accordance with the Good Clinical Practice (GCP) guidelines of the European Community.

3.3
Results

3.3.1
Bacterial Count

The results of the log-transformed counts are given in Table 3.2, those of the statistics in Table 3.3. The count of *Staphylococcus aureus* dropped by more than three orders of magnitude under mupirocin treatment and somewhat less under ciclopirox compared with the cream base and the untreated site. Whereas the negative controls nearly kept their initial counts in the case of *Staphylococcus aureus* pyoderma, in the case of *Streptococcus pyogenes* they

Table 3.2. Log_{10}-transformed bacterial counts (mean ± standard deviation) 24 h after start (day 1), at end of treatment (day 5) and 2 days thereafter (day 7)

Species	Day	Ciclopirox	Cream base	Mupirocin	Untreated
Staphylococcus aureus	1	4.44 ± 1.79	6.93 ± 0.40	3.12 ± 2.15	6.59 ± 1.51
	5	0.99 ± 1.65	3.89 ± 2.27	0.49 ± 1.12	3.34 ± 2.87
	7	0.00 ± 0.00	2.32 ± 2.60	0.15 ± 0.76	2.23 ± 2.60
Streptococcus pyogenes	1	1.31 ± 2.01	3.15 ± 3.04	1.32 ± 1.86	3.29 ± 3.02
	5	0.00 ± 0.00	0.26 ± 1.29	0.00 ± 0.00	0.24 ± 1.19
	7	0.00 ± 0.00	0.07 ± 0.35	0.00 ± 0.00	0.00 ± 0.00

Table 3.3. Bacterial counts – essential statistics of treatment differences

Contrast based on ANOVA	Estimate	95% CI	p value[a]
Staphylococcus aureus			
Ciclopirox – ciclopirox vehicle cream	–2.49	[–3.37; –1.61]	<0.0001
Mupirocin ointment – untreated control	–3.48	[–4.36; –2.60]	<0.0001
Ciclopirox vehicle cream – untreated	0.34	[–0.54; 1.22]	0.4439
Streptococcus pyogenes			
Ciclopirox – ciclopirox vehicle cream	–1.84	[–2.69; –1.00]	<0.0001
Mupirocin ointment – untreated control	–1.97	[–2.82; –1.12]	<0.0001
Ciclopirox vehicle cream – untreated	–0.14	[–0.99; 0.71]	0.7392

ANOVA, analysis of variance; CI, confidence interval
[a] Two-sided *p* value

decreased by roughly 3.5–4 orders of magnitude. Nevertheless, the log-count was reduced approximately two additional orders of magnitude under ciclopirox olamine and the positive control mupirocin. At end of the treatment, *Streptococcus pyogenes* could hardly be found whatever the treatment was, whereas the *Staphylococcus aureus* count was still higher in vehicle and untreated sites than in either of the drug-treated sites.

The estimates obtained from the ANOVA (i.e., adjusting for a subject effect) of the contrast ciclopirox olamine cream minus vehicle for the logarithm of the number of bacteria were –2.49 (*Staphylococcus aureus*) and –1.84 (*Streptococcus pyogenes*), respectively, in favor of ciclopirox olamine cream. Treatment differences in either pyoderma were statistically highly significant ($p<0.0001$), as was the subject effect in the *Streptococcus pyogenes* infection, whereas no subject effect could be found in *Staphylococcus aureus* pyoderma ($p=0.1451$). Altogether, the main criterion indicates that ciclopirox olamine is superior to the vehicle in reducing the number of these gram-positive bacteria.

The contrast mupirocin minus control, evaluated to assess the sensitivity of the pyoderma model, showed a highly significant superiority of mupirocin over the controls in either pyoderma ($p<0.001$). The contrast vehicle minus control was not statistically significant, indicating that there was no vehicle effect.

3.3.2
Scores

The evolution of clinical signs is shown in Figs. 1–9, and the essential statistics for the comparisons at the end of treatment are given in Table 3.4. The clinical signs differ in the two pyodermas and are therefore presented separately.

3.3.2.1
Staphylococcus aureus Pyoderma

Papulopustules (Fig. 3.1) are hardly formed in the infected areas themselves, but could be observed on the surrounding skin and were assessed there. Ci-

Table 3.4. Clinical signs – essential statistics of treatment differences

Type of pyoderma and clinical signs	Ciclopirox minus vehicle			Mupirocin minus untreated control			Vehicle minus untreated control		
	Estimate	95% CI	p value[a]	Estimate	95% CI	p value[a]	Estimate	95% CI	p value[a]
Staphylococcus aureus									
Erythema	1.00	[0.68; 1.32]	<0.0001	−0.71	[−1.03; −0.39]	<0.0001	−0.17	[−0.49; 0.15]	0.3033
Edema/infiltration	0.21	[−0.03; 0.45]	0.0898	−0.33	[−0.57; −0.09]	0.0075	−0.17	[−0.41; 0.07]	0.1731
Papulopustules	−0.71	[−1.02; −0.40]	<0.0001	−0.54	[−0.85; −0.23]	0.0008	0.25	[−0.06; −0.56]	0.1104
Crusts/scaling	−0.17	[−0.59; 0.26]	0.4349	−0.67	[−1.09; −0.24]	0.0025	0.04	[−0.38; 0.47]	0.8449
Pus	0.79	[0.37; 1.21]	0.0003	−0.63	[−1.04; −0.21]	0.0039	−0.42	[−0.83; 0.00]	0.0504
Streptococcus pyogenes									
Erythema	1.50	[1.14; 1.86]	<0.0001	−0.33	[−0.69; 0.03]	0.0692	0.17	[−0.19; 0.53]	0.3592
Edema/infiltration	0.29	[0.09; 0.50]	0.0056	−0.13	[−0.33; 0.08]	0.2248	−0.04	[−0.25; 0.16]	0.6844
Papulopustules	−0.33	[−0.62; −0.05]	0.0221	−0.50	[−0.78; −0.22]	0.0008	0.04	[−0.24; 0.33]	0.7707
Crusts/scaling	0.00	[−0.11; 0.11]	1.0000	−0.04	[−0.15; 0.07]	0.4627	0.04	[−0.07; 0.15]	0.4627

CI, confidence interval.
[a]Two-sided p value

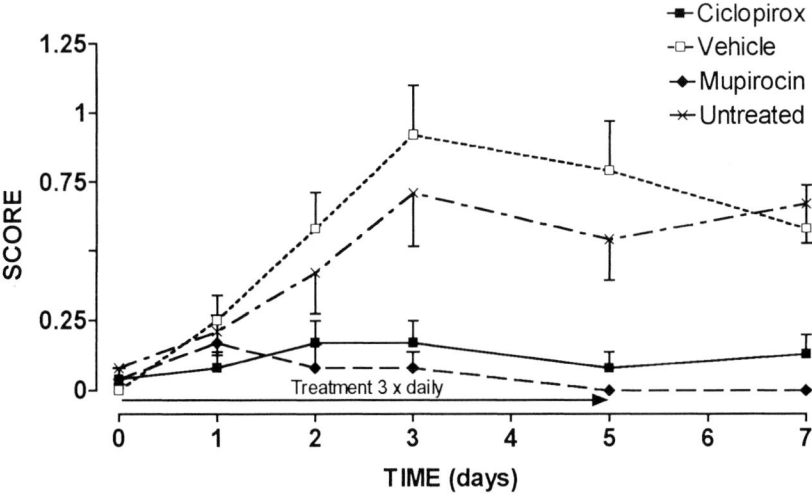

Fig. 3.1. Papulopustules on occluded skin surrounding the *Staphylococcus aureus* inoculation sites

clopirox was significantly better than the vehicle. Papulopustules on the surrounding occluded skin occurred rarely during the treatment course with ciclopirox olamine cream and were negligible under mupirocin cream, whereas they were obvious under the cream vehicle and the untreated control (ciclopirox olamine versus vehicle: $p<0.0001$ in the ANOVA, $p=0.00012$ in McNemar's test; mupirocin versus untreated control: $p=0.0008$).

A marginal superiority of ciclopirox olamine could also be found for *crusts/scaling* (Fig. 3.2). The maximum of these clinical signs at day 2 was lower for ciclopirox olamine cream (1.67±1.37) ($\bar{x}$±SD) relative to the vehicle (2.13±1.42) and the untreated control (2.13±1.30). However, crusts/scaling were similar at the end of treatment, regardless of whether the pyoderma was treated by ciclopirox olamine cream, its vehicle, or was left untreated, whereas it was less pronounced for the positive control.

The *erythema* score of the surrounding skin (Fig. 3.3) diminished only slightly under ciclopirox olamine treatment from 2.38±0.71 ($\bar{x}$±SD) at the start to 2.29±0.62 at the end of treatment and remained thereby significantly greater compared with the cream base (from 2.29±0.55 to 1.29±0.62) ($p<0.0001$). The erythema reduction during the treatment course was much more pronounced for the mupirocin cream (from 2.38±0.58 to 0.75±0.68) relative to the untreated control site (from 2.38±0.65 to 1.46±0.59) ($p<0.0001$).

The intensity of *edema/infiltration* (Fig. 3.4) diminished more under treatment with the two active drugs than with the vehicle and untreated control. Whereas mupirocin continued to return faster to normal than the untreated control ($p=0.0075$), the effect of ciclopirox olamine leveled off, leading even to a trend of somewhat greater signs for ciclopirox olamine relative to its vehicle at the end of the 5-day treatment period in the parametric analysis ($p=0.0989$). In the additional non-parametric test, no statistical difference

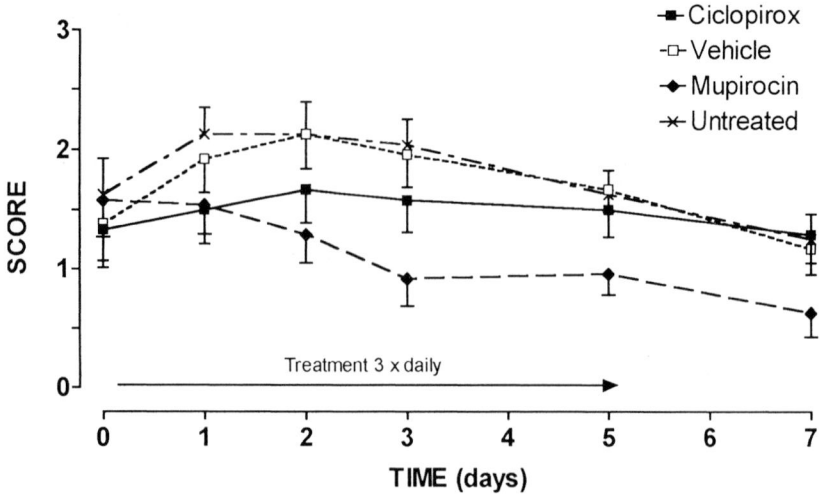

Fig. 3.2. Crusts/scaling on *Staphylococcus aureus* pyoderma sites

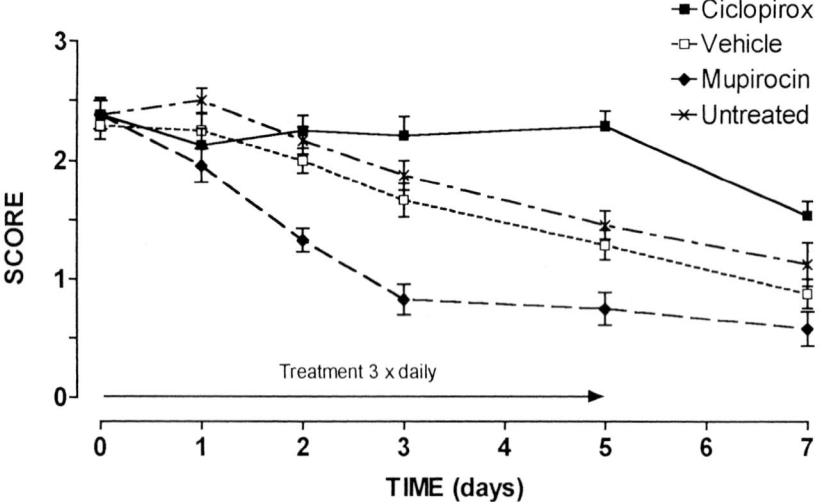

Fig. 3.3. Erythema induced by *Staphylococcus aureus* infection

could be found between ciclopirox olamine and the vehicle at that time point (one-sided $p=0.98047$).

Pus was a major clinical sign of *Staphylococcus aureus* pyoderma (Fig. 3.5). It was maximal after the inoculation period. The spontaneous regression strengthened at day 2, but was impeded by ciclopirox olamine at day 5 ($p=0.0003$), whereas it was enforced during the entire treatment period by mupirocin ($p=0.0039$).

No vehicle effect was observed at the end of treatment compared with the untreated control for any of the clinical signs (Table 3.4), except for pus for-

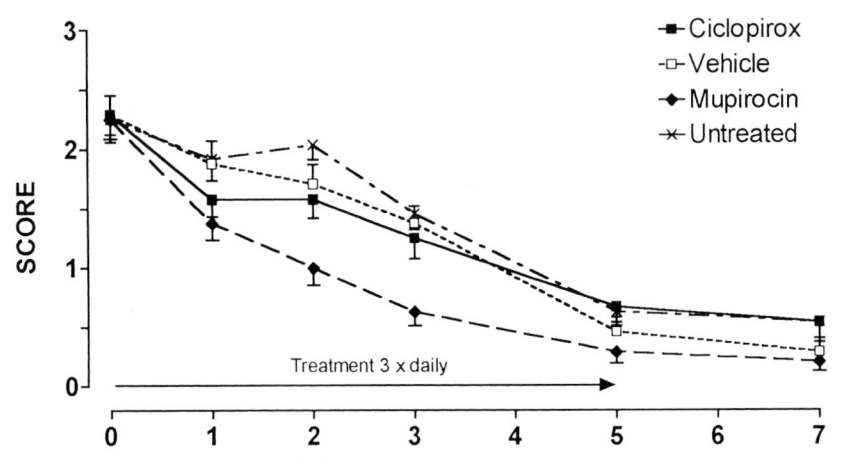

Fig. 3.4. Edema/infiltration of *Staphylococcus aureus* sites

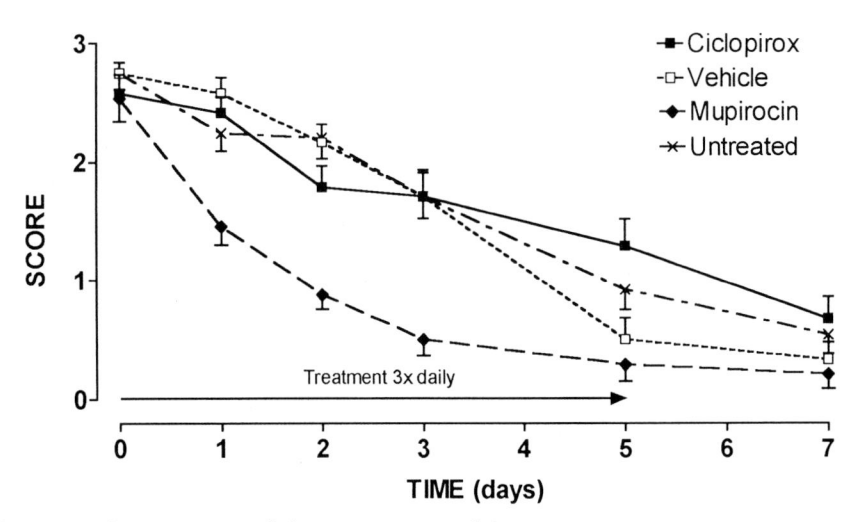

Fig. 3.5. Pus formation in *Staphylococcus aureus* pyoderma

mation, in which the greater reduction by the cream base nearly reached significance ($p=0.0504$).

3.3.2.2
Streptococcus pyogenes Pyoderma

Papulopustules were the hallmark of this type of pyoderma (Fig. 3.6). This sign diminished much faster under the two active treatments ($p=0.0221$ for ciclopirox olamine versus vehicle; $p=0.0008$ for mupirocin versus untreated control). Significant differences between ciclopirox olamine cream and its ve-

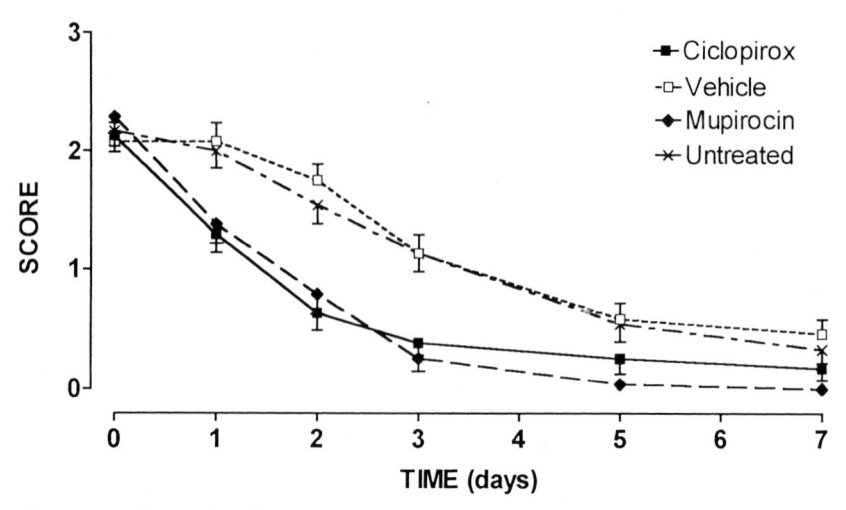

Fig. 3.6. Papulopustules of *Streptococcus pyogenes*-inoculated sites

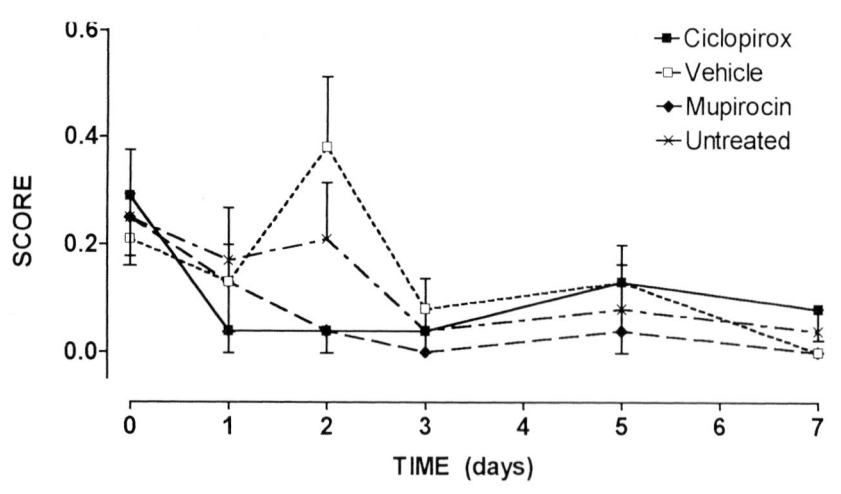

Fig. 3.7. Crusts/scaling in *Streptococcus pyogenes* pyoderma (note the maximum of the y-axis)

hicle could also be shown using the non-parametric McNemar's test ($p=0.01953$).

Crusts/scaling (Fig. 3.7) were only seen in some cases in the two negative controls with the maximum at day 2 of treatment.

Erythema (Fig. 3.8) diminished slowest under ciclopirox olamine cream and fastest under mupirocin cream, as could already be observed in *Staphylococcus aureus* pyoderma. The erythema remained significantly more pronounced under ciclopirox olamine cream treatment compared with its vehicle ($p=0.0001$), whereas the trend for a better treatment effect of mupirocin nearly reached significance compared with untreated control ($p=0.0692$).

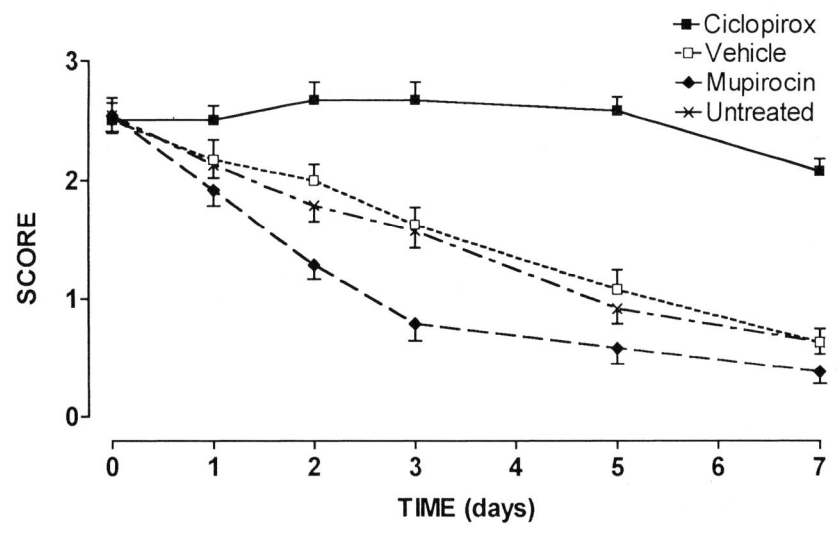

Fig. 3.8. Erythema in *Streptococcus pyogenes* infection

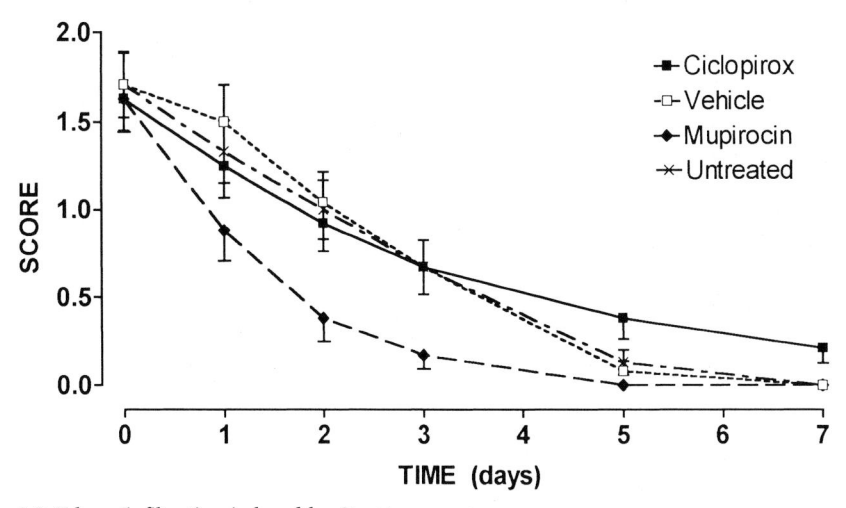

Fig. 3.9. Edema/infiltration induced by *Streptococcus pyogenes*

Edema/infiltration (Fig. 3.9) was not as developed in *Streptococcus pyogenes* infection as it was in *Staphylococcus aureus* pyoderma. At the end of treatment, only ciclopirox olamine cream-treated sites still showed some infiltration, which could even be seen 2 days thereafter, leading to an overall significant superiority of the vehicle ($p=0.0056$). These signs diminished fastest under mupirocin cream, but even the difference of the latter to untreated control was not significant ($p=0.2248$).

Pus was rarely seen in *Streptococcus pyogenes* infection (therefore not shown).

No vehicle effect was found at the end of treatment compared with the untreated control for any of the clinical signs (Table 3.4).

3.3.3
Adverse Events

No drug-related adverse event was observed except a contact dermatitis in one subject, which was very probably caused by ciclopirox olamine cream. An irritation potential by ciclopirox olamine under occlusive conditions will be discussed later. No hints were found for a systemic reaction to the experimental infections or the treatments.

3.4
Discussion

Ciclopirox olamine cream was an effective topical antimicrobial agent against two types of superficial pyodermas caused by the most common responsible pathogenic bacteria, *Staphylococcus aureus* and *Streptococcus pyogenes*. The bacterial counts were significantly further reduced by ciclopirox olamine cream within the first 24 h compared with the vehicle cream (*Staphylococcus aureus*: 2.5 orders of magnitude; *Streptococcus pyogenes*: nearly two orders of magnitude).

The reason why day 1 was taken for assessing the efficacy on bacterial counts was the known time course in naturally occurring as well as artificially induced diseases. Spontaneous reduction of the number of *Streptococcus pyogenes* is a regular finding even under occlusion, in contrast to *Staphylococcus aureus*, thereby decreasing the absolute differences in that type of pyoderma. This phenomenon usually leads to spontaneous disappearance of *Streptococcus pyogenes* within a few days, as could be seen by the bacterial count of the untreated control site at days 1, 5, and 7 in this study and as is known from the literature [7, 11]. The sites were inoculated by – a log-transformed number of – approximately 7.00 streptococci under occlusion, but had reduced 48 h later (day 1) to 3.29±3.02 at the untreated control sites and could hardly be detected anymore in those sites at the end of treatment (0.24±1.19), nor in any of the samples 2 days after stopping the occlusion. In contrast, the number of staphylococci was spontaneously diminished only at day 5 to roughly the same extent as streptococci at day 1. In consequence, antibiotic effects can more accurately be observed 1–2 days after the start of treatment, although the effect of the two active drugs was still evident at the end of treatment in the case of the staphylococcal pyoderma.

In order to interpret the clinical results obtained, it has to be taken into account that the two types of pyoderma differ in their spontaneous evolution and in their clinical appearance.

The hallmark of staphylococcal pyoderma was pus formation over the whole inoculated site and follicular papulopustules in the surrounding occluded skin, probably caused by some spreading of the infection, whereas papulopustules within the inoculated test sites were the major clinical sign of streptococcal pyoderma. Taking these major signs of either pyoderma, the clinical efficacy roughly corresponded to that of the bacterial counts. Mupirocin ointment used as a reference product was superior to the untreated control and at least equal to ciclopirox olamine cream in terms of bacteriological clearing. It was also best in terms of accelerating the clinical healing. The clinical efficacy of ciclopirox olamine cream could be shown by preventing spreading of *Staphylococcus aureus* (papulopustules on the surrounding skin) and by reducing the formation of crusts and scaling in *Staphylococcus aureus* pyoderma. The clinical benefit of ciclopirox olamine cream was also superior in the case of *Streptococcus pyogenes* infection relative to the cream base, since the hallmark in the form of papulopustules was more greatly reduced by the former.

There is a continuous debate about the risk/benefit ratio of topical antibiotics in treating pyoderma. The exclusive application of antibiotics topically for the treatment of bullous impetigo and widespread pyoderma is on the one hand regarded as professional malpractice [12], but on the other hand taken as useful as long as the lesions are not too widespread [13]. Such views reflect the wide range of pyodermic lesions and the difficulties in deciding what type of treatment is best, and thus correspond rather to opinions than proofs. It is not within the scope of this article to try to cover all the facets of this particular decision process. However, it seems justified to state that ciclopirox olamine is a good candidate for treating mixed infections such as athlete's foot.

The lack of pus formation in streptococcal infection was different from previous reports [7, 10, 11]. We used conditions similar if not identical to those previously described, and the inoculum was 2 orders of magnitude higher. Presumably the virulence of the strain was lower, although this strain was more virulent in pilot experiments than a T-3 strain (DSM 2074) probably one of the strains also used by Leyden et al. [7].

Erythema is a common sign in either pyoderma that should be reduced by the active drug treatments, but in fact it remained longer during and following the treatment by ciclopirox olamine relative to the negative controls (vehicle and untreated). The discrepancy between the good treatment effect on the number of bacteria and the corresponding main criterion of either pyoderma on the one hand and the much smaller clinical effect on some other clinical criteria on the other hand can be explained by an irritating effect. Irritation became obvious by the prolonged erythematous reaction in either pyoderma and in the case of *Staphylococcus aureus*, also by the prolonged pus formation compared with the other clinical signs.

Interpreting discrepancies in the evolution of the various clinical signs under ciclopirox olamine as irritation is supported by the finding that irritation was also observed in another study using ciclopirox olamine under occlusive conditions in experimentally induced dermatophytosis (in preparation). Ciclopirox olamine cream, but not the vehicle, induced mild irritation under the occlusive conditions used in this study in contrast to the usual unoccluded application, suggesting that ciclopirox olamine itself is responsible (already described in appendix B of the investigator's brochure as mild-to-moderate irritation).

A contact dermatitis was observed in one subject, which was probably caused by ciclopirox olamine cream. The small number of subjects in this study does not allow speculation about the sensitization rate. However, no important sensitization rate is known from a human sensitization assay or has became obvious during clinical use.

3.5 Conclusion

Antimicrobial as well as clinical efficacy of ciclopirox olamine cream was shown in the two most common types of pyoderma, i.e., superficial skin infections caused by *Staphylococcus aureus* and *Streptococcus pyogenes*.

The in vivo factors, in particular the inflammatory reaction leading to pus formation, crusts and scaling, do not abolish the drug's antimicrobial activity. Ciclopirox olamine is therefore a first candidate for mixed infections such as athlete's foot, since it has an antibiotic spectrum against gram-positive and gram-negative bacteria as well as antifungal activity. No relevant adverse events were observed beside the known irritant potential.

Acknowledgement. We thank Dr. Sauermann, DataMap GmbH, 79111 Freiburg, Germany, for the statistics and Dr. Witte, Robert-Koch-Institute, for providing the Staphylococcus areus strain after its skilful characterization.

References

1. Brandis H, Köhler W, Eggers HJ, Pulverer G (eds) (1994) Medizinische Mikrobiologie, 7. Aufl. Gustav Fischer, Stuttgart Jena New York
2. Burkhardt F (ed) (1992) Mikrobiologische Diagnostik. Thieme, Stuttgart New York
3. Davis B, Dulbecco R, Eisen HN, Ginsberg HS (eds) (1990) Microbiology, 4th edn. Lippincott, Philadelphia
4. Noble WC (1983) Microbial skin disease: its epidemiology. Edward Arnold, London
5. Rose NR, Barron AL, Crane LR, Menna JH (eds) (1983) Microbiology – basic principles and clinical applications. Macmillan, New York Toronto London
6. Werner H (ed) (1992) Medizinische Mikrobiologie mit Repetitorium. de Gruyter, Berlin, New York
7. Leyden JJ, Stewart R, Kligman AM (1980) Experimental infections with group A streptococci in humans. J Invest Dermatol 75:196–201
8. Frosch P, Kligman AM (1977) Rapid blister formation in human skin with ammonium hydroxide. Br J Dermatol 96:461–473
9. Williamson P, Kligman AM (1965) A new method for quantitative investigation of cutaneous bacteria. J Invest Dermatol 45:498–503
10. Singh G, Marples RR, Kligman AM (1971) Experimental *Staphylococcus aureus* infections in humans. J Invest Dermatol 57:149–162
11. Leyden JJ (1990) Mupirocin: a new topical antibiotic. J Am Acad Dermatol 22:879–883
12. Merk HF, Bickers DR (1992) Dermatopharmakologie und Dermatotherapie. Blackwell Wissenschaft, Berlin
13. Orfanos CE, Garbe C (1995) Therapie der Hautkrankheiten. Springer, Berlin

CHAPTER 4

Studies of the Anti-Inflammatory Properties of Ciclopirox

J. L. REES

There is considerable interest in the anti-inflammatory properties of ciclopirox. Many would argue that there would be a considerable niche for a product that had wide-ranging anti-infective properties but that could also inhibit the inflammatory response. The evidence for the anti-inflammatory activity of ciclopirox comes from a number of directions: clinical studies whose primary end points were concerned with antimycotic activity; limited studies of ultraviolet radiation-induced erythema in man; and inhibition of swelling following application of arachidonic acid to the mouse ear, as well as in vitro models of cellular production of PGE2 and 5-HETE (data on file). It is clearly desirable to investigate these properties further and critically review present results.

Assessment of anti-inflammatory activity based on clinical studies of seborrhoeic dermatitis is problematic, as the potent antimycotic activity of ciclopirox may confound any interpretation of anti-inflammatory activity in the clinical setting. On the other hand, the clinical predictive ability and utility of experimental in vivo experiments in the mouse, or a number of in vitro assays carried out to date for ciclopirox, is at present not clear. Nevertheless, the in vitro data are suggestive and warrant further investigation. Work to date has shown that following the application of arachidonic acid to the mouse ear, ciclopirox results in a >40% inhibition of oedema, similar to that seen for desometasone and indomethacin. By contrast, other anti-fungal agents such as fluconazole and ketoconazole show little activity, and some such as miconazole appear to actually increase oedema. In order to dissect out the putative mechanisms underlying these observations, in vitro studies have been performed examining the effects of ciclopirox on the inhibition of 5-lipoxygenase metabolite production (5-HETE and LTB4) and cyclooxygenase metabolite (PGE2) cellular release. Ciclopirox and ciclopirox olamine both show a striking inhibition of 5-HETE and LTB4 formation. Rilopirox also shows potent activity. By contrast, other clinically relevant comparable agents such as miconazole and ketoconazole show lower effects. Inhibition, however, of PGE2 cellular release is more modest, at around 25%, in comparison with indomethacin, scored as 100% change from control.

To date, experimental studies on man are limited. Ciclopirox has, however, been shown to inhibit ultraviolet radiation-induced erythema, with one study showing a 50% inhibition of erythema, comparable to the result obtained with hydrocortisone, and greater than any change seen with ketoconazole, miconazole, naftifine or amorolfine. Results for indomethacin within the same experiment were not available. There is therefore a need to extend these experimental studies and, because of the wide divergence and networking of inflammatory mediators involved in skin disease, a necessity to encompass a range of different assays reflecting different characteristics of the inflammatory response. We have therefore chosen to examine the effect of ciclopirox on a range of inflammatory model systems, namely inhibition of ultraviolet A and B erythema, inhibition of contact allergic eczema to dinitrochlorobenzene, inhibition of irritant contact eczema secondary to sodium dodecyl sulphate and inhibition of free radical-mediated (at least in part) anthralin-induced inflammation [1]. These studies are in their infancy, but a brief sketch of the methodology together with preliminary results on the inhibition of ultraviolet erythema are presented below.

4.1
Inhibition of Ultraviolet Erythema

Graded dose-responses using root 2 increments can be generated using monochromatic sources close to 300 nm on the backs of healthy volunteers. Inflammation can be assessed as a change in erythema using a reflectance instrument at various time points from 2–48 h after application of ciclopirox under occlusion following irradiation [1, 2]. The data can be statistically manipulated to produce characteristic dose-response curves, as described, allowing examination of agents that alter the threshold or the slopes of the resulting curves. Using this system, it is possible to pre-treat with the agent and, because the inflammatory pathways have different wavelengths, to use a range of different wavebands. We have carried out studies on eight subjects using a variety of strengths of ciclopirox under occlusion for 2 h and examined changes in erythema between 2 and 24 h. Results to date show clear differences from control in some individuals, although the pattern appears to be complex. Because of the preliminary nature of these experiments, we have examined at multiple different time points in different individuals; a consistent pattern has not been seen, however, and studies of a larger number of subjects and examination of multiple time points within any one individual are required. Studies using ultraviolet A are in progress.

We also propose to examine other models of inflammation, as discussed above. Anthralin can conveniently be applied in chloroform and modified Harpenden calipers used to assess changes in skin thickness as a proxy for a measure of inflammation. This system has been previously validated and shown to be sensitive to a variety of agents including corticosteroids and free radical scavengers [3]. Eczema, both irritant and allergic, is also amenable to quantitative study. Quantitative techniques for the assessment for contact allergic eczema secondary to dinitrochlorobenzene were developed in Newcastle using a fairly simple and straightforward methodology [4]. Graded doses applied to defined areas of skin on the upper inner arm or thigh can be used to sensitise individuals and then graded doses applied as a challenge 3–4 weeks later.

Again, the data are amenable to statistical analysis, producing dose-response curves that again can be analysed for differences in threshold and slope effects [4, 5]. Irritant dermatitis secondary to sodium dodecyl sulphate can also be studied by analogous methods using either erythema or water loss as an end point [6]. Current studies using these techniques with ciclopirox are in progress.

References

1. Farr PM, Lawrence CM, Shuster S (1989) Measurement of skin thickness, wealing, irritant, immune and ultraviolet response in skin. In: Greaves MW, Shuster S (eds) Pharmacology of the skin. Springer, Berlin, pp 55–62
2. Diffey BL, Farr PM (1991) Quantitative aspects of ultraviolet erythema. Clin Phys Physiol Meas 12:311–325
3. Finnen MJ, Lawrence CM, Shuster S (1991) Inhibition of dithranol inflammation by free-radical scavengers. Lancet 2:1129–1130
4. Friedman PS, Moss C (1985) Quantification of contact hypersensitivity in man. In: Maibach H, Lowe N (eds) Models in dermatology. Karger, Basel, pp 275–281
5. Rees JL, Matthews JN, Friedmann PS (1992) Quantifying anti-inflammatory agents' potency by measurement of response to dinitrochlorobenzene challenge. J Dermatol Sci 4:1–5
6. Cowley NC, Farr PM (1992) A dose-response study of irritant reactions to sodium lauryl sulphate in patients with seborrhoeic dermatitis and atopic eczema. Acta Derm Venereol. 72:432–435

CHAPTER 5

Measurement of Ciclopirox Permeation Through Fingernail Models by Novel Spectroscopic Techniques

T. M. BAYERL

Abstract

We have studied the permeation of ciclopirox through models of a fingernail, employing two new spectroscopic methods that were recently developed by our group. One is the measurement of permeation by means of infrared attenuated total reflection (IR)-ATR spectroscopy, the other is based on a specialized nuclear magnetic resonance (NMR) microscopy technique. Both methods indicate that topically applied ciclopirox solution penetrates through the fingernail and into the skin matrix.

5.1 Methods

The infrared spectroscopy approach is based on the ATR technique and allows the precise determination of all essential permeation parameters of a formulation, or of a single component, through a permeable layer (human skin, fingernail, etc.), without the need of any labelling of the molecules [1]. Additionally, it can provide detailed information on the possible metabolization of the permeant on its way through the layer. IR-ATR measurements of ciclopirox permeation were done as described in detail previously [1]. A 0.5-mm-thick cow horn plate of 2.0×0.5-cm size was placed on top of a horizontal silicon ATR plate. A rectangular teflon frame pressed the horn plate firmly to the ATR plate to ensure maximum contact area between the silicon surface and the bottom side of the horn plate. This allows the evanescent IR field emerging from the ATR crystal to penetrate about 1 µm deep into the bottom side of the horn plate facing the crystal. Thus, only those parts of the ciclopirox solution (8 mg in 1 ml isopropanol), applied topically on top of the 0.5-mm-thick horn plate, that manage to permeate through to the bottom of the plate will be detected by its fingerprint infrared signal. The permeation kinetics are then obtained by a time-resolved IR measurement and intensity analysis of the ciclopirox fingerprint IR bands.

The NMR method was applied for the non-invasive observation of the permeant passage through the layer, with focus on the skin below the fingernail.

Measurement of Ciclopirox Permeation Through Fingernail Models

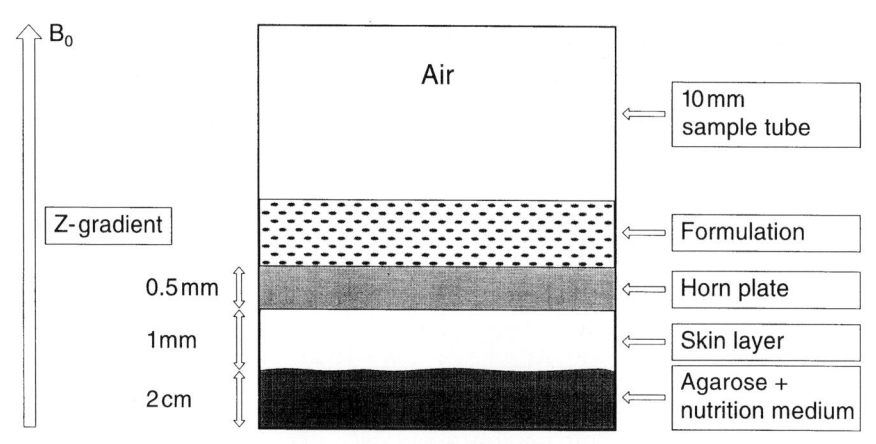

Fig. 5.1. Schematic depiction of the fingernail model setup used in the nuclear magnetic resonance (NMR) experiments (*left*) and a NMR spin-density microscopic image of the setup with ciclopirox solution on top of the horn plate at 100-μm resolution (*right*). The *arrow* indicates the direction of the magnetic field in the NMR magnet

The potential advantage of the NMR microscopy technique is that it allows a visualization of the instananeous permeant distribution in consecutive layers of ~50-μm thickness each. This resolution is sufficient to distinguish the skin stratum corneum from the lower (dermal) layers. Our fingernail model for the NMR microscopy was a circular, 1-mm-thick horn plate of 10-mm diameter on top of a circular piece (same diameter) of fresh human skin supported by an agar and enclosed by a cylindrical 10-mm NMR tube (Fig. 5.1). The ciclopirox solution was topically applied at the same concentration as for IR and a chemical shift imaging (CSI) pulse sequence [2] was used to visualize the ciclopirox on its way through the horn and into the skin below it. Figure 5.1 depicts the setup together with an NMR spin-density microscopic image of it.

5.2
Results and Discussion

Figure 5.2 shows the permeation kinetics of ciclopirox as determined by the IR-ATR technique. These results allow the estimation of a permeation half-time of several hours and show clearly that the permeant passes through the horn plate. The exact nature of the transport process that shuttles the rather hydrophobic ciclopirox though the porous horn plate is not yet known. We conjecture that the solvent is critical in this process and may serve as a surface diffusion mediator.

The NMR data confirm the IR results regarding the permeation of ciclopirox, but its visualization within the horn and the skin is hampered by a drastic decrease in the transverse relaxation time of the ciclopirox signals upon entering these layers and within them. In contrast, the less hydropho-

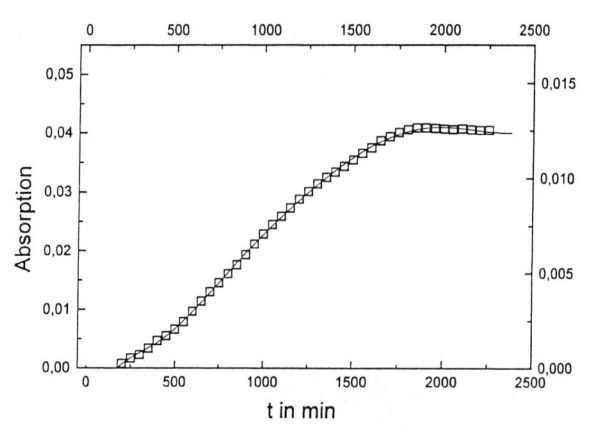

Fig. 5.2. Permeation kinetics of ciclopirox solution through human skin determined by time-resolved infrared attenuated total reflection (ATR) measurements

bic solvent (isopropanol) can be visualized at all points of its passage. Nevertheless, signals of both ciclopirox and isopropanol were observed in the gap between the bottom of the horn plate and the stratum corneum of the skin attached to it. This indicates that the invisibility of ciclopirox within the layer is indeed a technical problem owing to its solid-like relaxation behavior. We conclude that the NMR technique has high potential for the in vivo microscopic visualization of permeating substances, provided that the permeants are sufficiently hydrophilic to retain a high degree of molecular mobility at all stages of the permeation process.

References

1. Reinl H, Hartinger A, Dettmar P, Bayerl TM (1995) Time resolved infrared ATR measurements of liposome transport kinetics in human keratinocyte cultures and skin reveals a dependence on liposome size and phase state. J Invest Dermatol 105:291–295
2. Kwon-Song H, Wehrli FW, Ma J (1997) In vivo MR microscopy of the human skin. Magn Reson Med 37:185–191

CHAPTER 6

Dermatomycosis: A Multifactorial Disease

M. A. J. ALLEVATO

Superficial mycoses (dermatomycoses) occur all over the world; they are one of the most frequent infections of mankind. The World Health Organization considers that 20% of the world population suffers from superficial mycosis, and this percentage is even higher in tropical and subtropical areas. Most of these infections are caused by dermatophytes (dermatophytosis), and they involve the skin, the hair, and the nails. There are also two types of cutaneous infections caused by yeasts. *Candida* species, usually *Candida albicans*, cause infections of the mucous membrane, skin and fingernails, whereas *Malassezia furfur* infects the skin, usually the trunk (pityriasis versicolor).

Although some of these infections have a typical clinical picture, some cases may lead to misdiagnosis with other non-mycotic skin diseases. The clinical picture depends on multiple factors, the most relevant of which are the host, the pathogen, the skin area, and the geographic area. Without doubt, the host-pathogen relation should be stressed, as in any infectious disease, whether of mycotic or other origin.

The host factor (Table 6.1) plays a major role in the development of most fungal infections. Different epidemiologic studies indicate the existence of a genetic susceptibility to superficial mycoses.

A recent study conducted by Zaias and collaborators from Europe, the United States, and Argentina [13] showed that patients with distal subungual onychomycosis (DSO) appear to have a susceptibility to *Trichophyton rubrum* in a dominant autosomal pattern. All patients initially harbor *T. rubrum* in childhood, in the thick skin on the soles of the feet. From this early plantar tinea pedis, whose severity depends on individual factors, the infection can spread to other sites, producing other clinical signs of infection. It can, for instance, extend to the toenail (DSO), the groin (tinea cruris), the body skin (tinea corporis), or the palms and fingernails. These various expressions occur within a clinical syndrome that begins and remains chronic on the feet.

Other epidemiologic studies lend support to the view that pityriasis versicolor also occurs in patients with a genetic susceptibility.

Acquired factors may favor, perpetuate, or modify dermatomycoses in a wide variety of ways. The use of topical or systemic drugs may alter the saprophytic flora, as do antibiotics, or they may alter immunity, as do corticosteroids and cytostatic agents. In diseases such as diabetes and atopy, the incidence of dermatomycoses is higher, and it is also on the increase. Moreover, dermatomycoses in these diseases tend to be more extensive and more refractory to treatment.

Table 6.1. The host factor

Genetic susceptibility	Acquired factors	
• Dermatophytosis • Pityriasis versicolor • Candidosis	Drugs: General diseases: Occupational diseases Microtraumatism	Immunity alterations Flora alteration • Diabetes • Peripheral vascular diseases • AIDS • Other immunological diseases • Atopy

Circulatory alterations, especially in the lower extremities, produce visible skin modifications, which increase the incidence of mycotic infections. It is important to consider this modification when using oral antifungal agents, since their activity may be altered by the circulatory impairment.

Microtraumatisms owing to shaving of the legs may favor dermatomycoses in women. Women's toenails are also susceptible to microtraumata caused by shoes designed more for fashion than feet and/or orthopedic alterations.

The identification of the pathogen (Table 6.2) helps in understanding the clinical manifestations. As regards dermatomycoses, it is well known that microorganisms, whether zoophilic or geophilic, usually produce a strong inflammatory reaction. The dermatomycoses are contagious and spread by direct or indirect contact with an infected individual or animal. The infective particle is usually a fragment of keratin containing live fungus. In general, it is dermatophytes that cause these diseases. Different species of dermatophytes have adapted so as to cause infection in particular mammalian species. Furthermore, they have developed an affinity for particular types of keratin. Both these aspects are undoubtedly related to the types and quantities of proteolytic or keratinolytic enzymes they produce. These predilections have consequences for the pattern of infections seen in human beings, the varying risk of exposure in different environments, and the severity of the lesions caused.

In developed countries, the most prevalent form of dermatophytosis is foot ringworm (tinea pedis, athletes foot), with its associated infection of the nails, groin, and hands. It is mainly spread through the use of communal bathing places such as showers, saunas, and swimming pools. In the United Kingdom, for example, it is estimated that around 15% of the population has foot ringworm and 3–5% has nail dermatophytosis. In certain groups who use communal bathing places frequently, such as industrial workers and coal miners, the prevalence of foot ringworm may be as high as 60–80%. The incidence of foot ringworm in the general population is likely to rise with the increased availability and use of sports and leisure centers that have communal bathing and shower facilities. Little effort is currently being made to control the spread of these infections.

Candida is a member of the commensal flora of human beings, and candidal infections are therefore mainly endogenous in origin; the exception is sexually transmitted genital candidosis. The carriage of *Candida* at different

Table 6.2. Identification of the pathogen

• Dermatophytes	– Anthropophilic – Zoophilic – Geophilic
• Malassezia (pityriasis versicolor)	
• Candida	

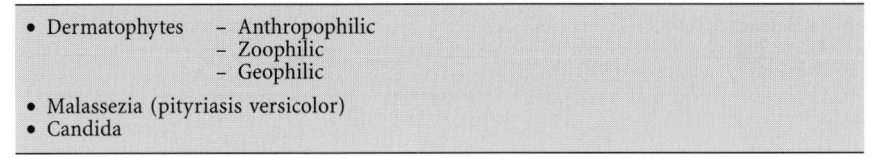

Table 6.3. The cutaneous anatomic area

• Skin	– Dry (folds) – Wet (foot/hand) – Sweating (groin): pityriasis versicolor
• Hair	Tinea
• Nails	Distal subungual onychomycosis Proximal subungual onychomycosis White superficial onychomycosis Candidosis

sites in different groups has been much studied; the results obtained have varied considerably depending on the population examined and the sampling methods used. We are now beginning to understand some of the factors that determine whether or not an individual harbors the organism. Local conditions play an important part, as does the ability of the organism to adhere to epithelial cells, which in turn is related to antigens and receptor sites both on the yeast and on the host cell surface. What causes commensal yeasts to become pathogenic is still not well understood. Some of the factors identified as predisposing yeast to overgrowth and consequently causing infection may not actually do so; and even if they do, the mechanism involved may not necessarily be the one previously supposed. Much work has been done on the source of *Candida* and the routes by which it spreads, particularly in relation to problems such as recurrent vaginal candidosis.

Epidemiological studies of this kind have become more meaningful since the introduction of methods for the DNA typing of *Candida* isolates. A better understanding of the epidemiology of candidosis will allow the introduction of improved prophylaxis regimes for patients exposed to the risk of *Candida* infection.

Pityriasis versicolor infections are also thought to be endogenous in origin, with the causal agent *M. furfur* (*Pityrosporon ovale*) being found on the skin and scalp of a large proportion of the normal population. What induces the yeast to become pathogenic and cause the disease pityriasis versicolor is not clearly understood, although high temperatures and humidity may play a role, since the disease is much prevalent in tropical and subtropical parts of the world, where it is often the most common superficial mycosis.

The cutaneous anatomic area (Table 6.3) may determine different degrees of susceptibility to dermatomycoses. Undoubtedly, wet and traumatized areas will be more prone.

In onychomycosis, it is important to consider the increase in the proximal subungual form in patients with AIDS.

Table 6.4. Geographic area

- Climate: dermatomycoses occur mainly in tropical and subtropical areas
- Agent: prevalence varies according to species
- Host: socio-cultural and dietary habits

The geographic area (Table 6.4) is another factor to be considered, since it is well known that tropical and subtropical climates favor dermatomycoses. Variation in the prevalence of pathogens from region to region is important when evaluating the clinical expression and therapeutic approach. For example, in Argentina, the cases of tinea owing to *Trichophyton tonsurans* are not frequent. Dressing, dietary, and hygiene habits also contribute to the development of this disease.

To summarize, dermatomycosis is a multifactorial disease, and all the factors involved are in a continuous state of change. We have to be fully aware of this if we are to identify and understand them.

References

1. Baran R, Badillet G (1983) Un dermatophyte ungueal est-il necessairement pathogene? Ann Dermatol Venereol 110:629–631
2. Binazzi M, Papini M, Simonetti S (1983) Skin mycoses – geographic distribution and present day pathomorphosis. Int J Dermatol 22:92–97
3. Caprilli F, Mercantini R, Polamava G, et al (1986) Distribution and frequency of dermatophytes in the city of Rome between 1978 and 1983. Mykosen 30:86–93
4. Greer DL (1995) The evolving role of nondermatophytes in onychomycosis. Int J Dermatol 34:521–524
5. Korstanje MJ, Staats CC (1995) Fungal infections in the Netherlands. Prevailing fungi and pattern of infection. Dermatology 190:39–42
6. Macura AB (1995) Dermatophytes: pathogens or saprophytes. Int J Dermatol 34:529–530
7. Odom R (1993) Pathophysiology of dermatophyte infections. J Am Acad Dermatol 28:52–57
8. Pereiro Miguens M, Pereiro M, Pereiro M Jr (1991) Review of dermatophytoses in Galicia from 1951 to 1987 and comparision with other areas of Spain. Mycopathologia 113:65–78
9. Rippon JW (1992) Forty-four years of dermatophytes in a Chicago clinic (1944–1988). Mycopathologia 119:25–28
10. Svejgaard E (1986) Epidemiology and clinical features of dermatomycoses and dermatophytoses. Acta Derm Venereol Suppl (Stockh) 121:19–26
11. Svejgaard E (1995) Epidemiology of dermatophytes in Europe. Int J Dermatol 34:525–528
12. Torres-Rodriguez JM, Balaguer-Meler J, Ventin-Hernandez M, et al (1986) Multicenter study of dermatophyte distribution in the metropolitan area of Barcelona (Catalonia, Spain). Mycopathologia 93:95–97
13. Zaias N, Tosti A, Rebell G, Morelli R, Bardazzi F, Beilley H, Zaiac M, Glick B, Paley B, Allevato M, Baran R (1996) Autosomal dominant pattern of distal subungual onychomycosis caused by *Trichophyton rubrum*. J Am Acad Dermatol 34:302–304

CHAPTER 7

Efficacy of Topical Batrafen

S. A. Burova

7.1
Introduction

Although superficial fungal infections rarely involve the morbidity and mortality seen with systemic infections such as candidiasis, aspergillosis and criptococcal infections, they constitute a common health problem of increasing incidence.

Candida is a classic opportunistic pathogen, and candidiasis is a common infection. There are many sites susceptible to *Candida* infections. Examples are *Candida granuloma* of the scalp, oral candidiasis, intertriginous candidiasis of major flexures, and interdigital candidiasis. Even in transient and trivial local infections, predisposing factors such as obesity, moisture and maceration, diabetes, pregnancy, the use of the contraceptive pill and broad-spectrum antibiotics often play a significant part in development of the disease.

In our clinical study, the efficacy of Batrafen (ciclopiroxolamine) cream was investigated in patients with *Candida* infections of the skin. Batrafen (Hoechst) has antifungal and antibacterial activity in vitro against *Candida spp.*, *Trichophyton spp.*, *Microsporum spp.*, *Aspergillus spp.*, *Penicillium spp.*, gram-positive bacteria, gram-negative bateria, and microplasma.

7.2
Methods

Of the 14 patients studied, seven were suffering from chronic cutaneous candidiasis, four patients from *Candida intertrigo* and three patients from chronic paronychia. *Candida albicans* was identified as the pathogen in all 14 patients. Before treatment, the diagnosis was confirmed by clinical pictures and cultivation tests. The duration of infection ranged from 8–12 weeks. The mean age was 38 years (range 17–62); four patients were male and ten female.

Medical histories were recorded and physical examinations performed prior to treatment. Predisposing factors were recorded (Table 7.1).

Batrafen (ciclopirox) 1.0% cream was used twice a day topically. The duration of treatment was 8–10 days for four patients with *C. intertrigo*, 14–17 days for seven patients with chronic cutaneous candidiasis and 20–22 days for three patients with chronic paronychia.

Table 7.1. Predisposing factors

Diagnosis	Patient (n)	Predisposing factors				
		Pregnancy	Previous use of antibiotics	Diabetes	Obesity	Low serum iron
Chronic cutaneous candidiasis	7	3	2	1	2	1
Candida intertrigo	4	–	4	1	–	–
Chronic paronychia	3	2	1	2	–	1
Total	14	5	7	4	2	2

Table 7.2. Clinical and mycological response to therapy with Batrafen cream 1.0% in 14 patients with cutaneous candidiasis

Variable clinical	n	%
Patients evaluated	14	100
Response		
Cure	11	78.6
Improvement	2	14.3
Failure	1	7.1
Mycological patients	14	100
Response		
Eradication	12	85.7
Failure	2	14.3

Signs and symptoms of the candidal infection were graded separately for each site of infection. Sites were categorised as chronic cutaneous candidiasis (neck, axilla, hands, trunk, groin), *C. intertrigo*, and chronic paronychia. Signs (scaling, vesicles, fissuring, maceration, erythema, rash and cellulitis) and symptoms (pruritus and burning) of candidiasis were recorded every 7 days during treatment and at the end of treatment. Scrapings were obtained from each site for myoclogical examination.

Patients were evaluated for safety at all review visits. The criterion for clinical cure was the disappearance of the signs and symptoms described above. Improvement was defined as partial relief from or alleviation of signs and symptoms, and treatment failure was defined as no appreciable change in signs and symptoms. Clinical and mycological response is shown.

7.3
Results

As shown in Table 7.2, clinical cure was achieved in 11 cases, improvement in two cases, and failure was noted in one case. Mycological eradication was achieved in 12 cases. The results of this small study suggest that Batrafen cream 1% is an effective and safe drug for various types of cutaneous candidiasis.

CHAPTER 8

Ciclopirox Gel Treatment of Scalp Seborrheic Dermatitis

B. B. ABRAMS, R. J. CHERILL, R. RAMASWAMY and H. I. KATZ

Presented in part at:
"Hydroxy-Pyridones as Antifungal Agents", 23 May 1996, Vancouver, British Columbia, Canada.

The Ciclopirox Gel, Seborrheic Dermatitis Study Group.
R. Alky, San Francisco, CA; R. Berger, East Brunswick, NJ; D. Gorsulowsky, Fremont, CA; J. Hanifin, Portland OR; G. Izuno, La Jolla, CA; H. I. Katz, Minnesota Clinical Study Center, Fridley, MN; D. Lookingbill, S. Milton, Hershey Medical Center, Hershey, PA; N. Lowe, Santa Monica, CA; A. Menter, Texas Dermatology Associates, Dallas, TX; M. Morman, The Columns, Rutherford, NJ; D. Pariser, Virginia Clinical Research Center, Norfolk, VA; H. Roth, Daly City, CA; R. Savin, Savin Dermatology Center, PC, New Haven, CT; J. Shavin, Twinnett Clinical, Research Center, Snellville, GA; D. Stewart, Midwest Cutaneous Research, Clifton Township, MI; G. Webster, Thomas Jefferson University, Philadelphia, PA.

8.1
Introduction

Seborrheic dermatitis, a specific inflammatory dermatosis involving the scalp, face and chest, and dandruff, its minor form, have been attributed to *Pityrosporum ovale*, a yeast fungal organism [1–3]. The purpose of this paper is to describe the results of a multicenter study using topical ciclopirox gel 0.77% for the treatment of seborrheic dermatitis of the scalp.

8.2
Methods

Two similar studies, one with primarily scalp involvement and one with primarily facial involvement were conducted in patients with seborrheic dermatitis. Both studies were randomized, double-blind, vehicle-controlled, and multicenter. Prior to initiation of the study, at each investigative site, institutional board approval of the protocol and informed consent were obtained.

Participants provided both verbal and written informed consents. Key baseline inclusion criteria were:
1. Age > 18 years
2. Seborrheic dermatitis of face or scalp
3. Total score of at least 4 for pruritus, burning, erythema and/or scale 0–3 for each sign of symptom
4. Signed informed consent
5. Female patients of child-bearing potential
6. Use birth control method(s)

The exclusion criteria were as follows:
1. Pregnant or nursing female patients
2. Psoriasis, atopic dermatitis, acne, or rosacea
3. Uncontrolled diabetes, known HIV-positive or immunosuppressed subjects
4. Neurological disorders requiring treatment
5. Pre-baseline or concurrent potentially confounding topical or systemic medications such as: corticosteroids, antifungals, antibiotics or other anti-inflammatory medications

A mandatory 1-week pre-treatment washout was required for all patients, during which shampoo and facial soap use were standardized. Subjects were encouraged to keep their personal hygiene regimen unchanged during the study. Study test material, either ciclopirox gel or vehicle alone, was applied twice a day for up to 4 weeks. Return visits were made on days 4, 8, 15, 22 and 29. The primary efficacy variable was the global evaluation of scalp, improvement relative to baseline, evaluations of which were made at each follow-up visit, using a 6-point scale (0–5).

The severity of erythema, scaling, pruritus, and burning were rated separately in a representative scalp target area at each visit, using a scale that ranged from 0 = none, to 3 = severe (including half values, e.g., 2.5).

Efficacy analyses were performed only on data from the intent-to-treat population with qualifying scalp involvement at baseline, whereas safety analyses used the data from all patients.

8.3
Results

One-hundred-and-seventy-two subjects were randomized to treatment with ciclopirox gel and 173 subjects to treatment with the gel vehicle in the two studies combined (Table 8.1). Completion rates in the two groups were similar (>85%) in both studies. Demographic (Table 8.2) and baseline characteristics (Table 8.3) were similar for both groups, except that the vehicle treatment group had more subjects with an overall severity rating of severe, which necessitated an analytical p value adjustment (Tables 8.4, 8.5, below).

Efficacy analyses from both studies demonstrated a significantly greater improvement of scalp seborrheic dermatitis from ciclopirox gel than its vehicle. The mean global scores after both 2 weeks' treatment and end point

Table 8.1. Disposition of study cohort (pooled scalp and face results protocols 360 and 361)

	Ciclopirox	Vehicle
Randomized at baseline (n)	172	173
Completed study	151 (88%)	147 (85%)
Did not complete study	21 (12%)	26 (15%)
Lack of efficacy	9 (5%)	13 (8%)
Adverse event	7 (4%)	7 (4%)
Other reasons	5 (3%)	6 (3%)

Table 8.2. Demographics of study participants with qualifying scalp seborrheic dermatitis only

	Ciclopirox	Vehicle
n	132	133
Sex	83 male; 49 female	97 male; 36 female
Race	117 white; 15 non-white	119 white; 14 non-white
Age (years), mean	45.5 ± 15.9	44.4 ± 15.2
Range (years)	(18–65)	(17–65)

Table 8.3. Baseline scalp seborrheic dermatitis status data

Overall severity	Ciclopirox (n)	Vehicle (n)
Total	132	133
Mild	25	25
Moderate	95	84
Severe	12	24
Disease duration		
>6 months	128	132
<6 months	4	1

showed moderate-to-excellent improvement (mean score 1.6) in the ciclopirox group compared with slight-to-moderate improvement (mean score 2.2) in the vehicle group (Table 8.4). The percentage change in the individual sign and symptom scores corresponded to the global scores (Table 8.5).

The incidence and severity of local adverse effects were similar to ciclopirox and vehicle (Table 8.6). The most frequent adverse effects were sensations of transient skin-burning on application, and irritant contact dermatitis. Most of these adverse effects occur on the face.

8.4
Discussion

Seborrheic dermatitis is a common relapsing subacute or chronic superficial inflammatory dermatosis that affects the scalp (including as its minor form, dandruff), face, and certain areas of the chest and back. The rash has a char-

Table 8.4. Mean global improvement scores

Mean global improvement scores[a]	n	Ciclopirox	Vehicle	Adjusted p value[b,c]
Day 4	125	2.9	3.1	0.361
Day 8	126	2.5	2.5	0.868
Day 15	124	2.1	2.4	0.037
Day 22	119	1.6	2.2	<0.001
Day 29	117	1.4	2.0	<0.001
End point	130	1.6	2.3	<0.001

[a] Global improvement scores: 0 = cleared, 100% clearance of disease; 1 = excellent improvement, 75–<100% clearance of disease; 2 = moderate improvement, 50–<75% clearance of disease; 3 = slight improvement, >0–<50% clearance of disease; 4 = no change, no improvement from baseline evaluation; 5 = exacerbation, flare of treatment area.
[b] Adjusted p value is a p value from rank analysis of covariance adjusted for disease severity.
[c] P value is from Mantel-Haenszel test (two tailed)

Table 8.5. Mean percentage change from baseline combined sign and symptom scores

Change mean score[a]	n	Ciclopirox	Vehicle	Adjusted p value[b,c]
Day 4	125	27.8	24.9	0.124
Day 8	126	43.4	42.4	0.207
Day 15	124	51.6	44.6	0.002
Day 22	119	65.6	50.6	<0.001
Day 20	117	72.3	57.8	<0.001
End point	130	63.8	51.2	<0.001

[a] Combined total scores for erythema, scaling, pruritus, and burning were rated using a scale that ranged from 0 (= none) to 3 (= severe). Half values, e.g., 2.5, could be used.
[b] Adjusted p value is a p value from rank analysis of covariance adjusted for disease severity.
[c] The p value is from Mantel-Haenszel test (two tailed)

Table 8.6. Local cutaneous adverse experiences that may be related to the study medication (pooled results protocols 360 and 361)

	Ciclopirox ($n=172$)	Vehicle ($n=173$)
Burning sensation	53	40
Application site reaction	6	3
Contact dermatitis	6	6
Pruritus	4	5
Dry skin	3	3
Acne	2	1
Alopecia	1	1
Rash	1	1

acteristic appearance with pruritus, erythema, and scale as its principal features. Seborrheic dermatitis and dandruff, its minor form have been attributed to *P. ovale* (*Malassezia furfur*) organisms [1-3]. While there are no permanent cures for seborrheic dermatitis, many of the established older treatments used to control seborrheic dermatitis and dandruff have been shown to have an antipityrosporal action [1-5]. Ketoconazole, a potent antipityrosporal agent was therefore selected for study and shown to be an effective treatment for seborrheic dermatitis [1, 2, 6-8]. Agents such as topical corticosteroid preparations have also been used to treat seborrheic dermatitis, but while their anti-inflammatory effect alleviates the condition, continued use leads to atrophy and telangiectasia and rosaeiia on the face.

Ciclopirox is a hydroxypyridinone antifungal agent, which may act by chelation of polyvalent cations; it has also been shown to have anti-inflammatory activity, and inhibits enzymes in the arachandonic acid cascade [9]. The olamine salt of ciclopirox has been marketed in various formulations in the United States and worldwide for more than 10 years. Its antipityrosporal effect suggests its suitability for seborrheic dermatitis, including its minor form, dandruff.

The results of the present studies demonstrate that ciclopirox gel 0.77% was significantly more effective than its vehicle in the treatment of seborrheic dermatitis of the scalp. A relatively high "placebo" response can occur in this condition and is presumed to be, in part, the inhibitory effect of vehicle on the *Pityrosporum* yeast. Adverse effects were not a problem; the most frequent was a transient burning sensation that occurred in 31% of patients. This reaction is probably owing to the alcohol content of the gel and is commonly experienced following applications of other alcohol-containing products such as after-shave lotions.

As with ketoconazole, the only prescription form of topical antifungal agent currently approved for the treatment of seborrheic dermatitis, and unlike topical corticosteroids, the response to ciclopirox requires a few weeks to be noticeable. However, seborrheic dermatitis is a chronic disorder, and repeated application of corticosteroids will produce unwanted effects. Thus, treatment with antipityrosporal agents such as ciclopirox is more appealing in acting directly on the causal agent and without a major potential for side effects.

8.5
Conclusion

The results of two randomized, vehicle-controlled, double-blind, parallel-group, multicenter studies demonstrate that ciclopirox gel, applied b.i.d. for up to 4 weeks, is an effective and safe therapy for the treatment of seborrheic dermatitisof the scalp.

Acknowledgement. This work was supported by a grant from Hoechst Marion Roussel, Inc., Somerville, N.J.

References

1. Shuster S (1984) The aetiology of dandruff and the mode of action of therapeutic agents. Br J Dermatol 111:235–242
2. Shuster S, Blatchford N (1988) Seborrhoeic dermatitis and dandruff – a fungal disease. (Congress & Symposium Series, vol 132) Royal Soc Med, London
3. Faergemann J (1994) *Pityrosporum* infections. J Am Acad Dermatol 31:S18–20
4. McGrath J, Murphy GM (1991) The control of seborrhoeic dermatitis and dandruff by antipityrosporal drugs. Drugs 41:178–184
5. Sei Y, Hamaguchi T, Ninomiya J, Nakabayashi A, Takiuchi I (1994) Seborrhoeic dermatitis; treatment with anti-mycotic agents. J Dermatol 21:334–340
6. Peter RU, Korting HC (1991) Treatment of seborrhoeic eczema with ketoconazole in comparison with an active agent-free cream (in German). Arzneimittelforschung 41:852–854
7. Danby FW, Maddin WS, Margesson LJ, Rosenthal D (1993) A randomized, double-blind, placebo-controlled trial of ketoconazole 2% shampoo versus selenium sulfide 2.5% shampoo in the treatment of moderate to severe dandruff. J Am Acad Dermatol 29:1008–1012
8. Peter RU, Richarz-Barthauer U (1995) Successful treatment and prophylaxis of scalp seborrhoeic dermatitis and dandruff with 2% ketoconazole shampoo: results of a multicentre, double-blind, placebo-controlled trial. Br J Dermatol 132:441–445
9. Abrams BB, Haenel H, Hoehler T (1991) Ciclopirox olamine; a hydroxypyridone antifungal agent. Clin Dermatol 9:471–477

CHAPTER 9

Seborrhoeic Dermatitis and Dandruff, and Its Treatment With Ciclopirox Shampoo

S. SHUSTER

9.1 Introduction – The Definition of Dandruff and Seborrhoeic Dermatitis as a Pityrosporal Infection

This chapter gives an account of the use of 1% ciclopirox shampoo in the treatment of seborrhoeic dermatitis of the scalp – which includes dandruff, its minor manifestation – and I will begin by explaining the rationale of this new therapy.

Like all simple things, the background was much complicated by an overgrowth of trivia, which was not cleared away until the summer of 1982, with the definitive definition of *Pityrosporum ovale* as the cause of dandruff. This reinstated that scaly disorder as crown prince to the empire of seborrhoeic dermatitis [1, 2] and gave a head start to its treatment.

In fact, the pityrosporum was first described by Rivolta in 1873 [3]. My guess (and, even if it is wrong, it is entertaining to entertain it) is that Rivolta found the organism when he was idly picking at a patch of seborrhoeic dermatitis growing in his beard, which he had misdiagnosed as psoriasis. It was in the following year that Malassez [4] first related the presence of the organism to "simple dandruff". But at that time, dandruff and seborrhoeic dermatitis were not well defined clinically; moreover, microbial attributions were becoming so common that the harsh scientific rationalisms of Robert Koch had to be introduced to calm the turbulent aetiological air. It is not surprising, therefore, that unsupported attributions such as those of Malassez were taken no more seriously than are present-day sightings of Unidentified Flying Objects. With such a flaccid background, it is also not surprising that, despite several tentative revisitings to the pityrosporal organism and its possible causal relationship to dandruff and seborrhoeic dermatitis, the idea of an aetiological relationship never prospered and, indeed, was generally dismissed.

And so, after years of jostling in a clinico-therapeutic void, dandruff and seborrhoeic dermatitis, the non-identical pityrosporal twins, became separated, as I have described elsewhere [5]. Seborrhoeic dermatitis was considered to be an eczematous reaction, and when the magic of topical corticosteroids became available, they became the appropriate treatment. It took time, the Til Eulenspiegel of accepted truth, to demonstrate the poverty of corticosteroid therapy: ever higher potencies were required for treatment, and the appearances of atrophy, telangiectasia and rosacea were added to the underlying rash. By contrast, dandruff was taken up more and more by the cosmetic industry than by dermatologists, and the culmination of the little research that was done on it, mostly in the 1960s and early 1970s, was believed to have established dandruff firmly as a hyperproliferative disease unrelated to the pityrosporum [6]. Indeed, the Food and Drug Administration (FDA) recommendations for antidandruff treatments specifically affirmed their antiproliferative, cytostatic mechanism, and these recommendations remained in place until the early 1980s.

What happened then might seem pure accident but, in fact, was the manipulation of serendipity, a scientific tool with which I have an abiding affinity. With various colleagues in the Department of Dermatology in Newcastle, I had been working for more years than was decent on the physiology of the sebaceous glands. Over these many years we had, to a very large extent, defined their endocrine and non-endocrine control in man and rat [6, 7] and then moved on to the obvious extension of sebaceous function in the production and actions of pheromones concerned with territorial marking, behaviour and sexual activity in gerbils, rats and mice [7]. What then happened was the social disaster of Thatcherite economies, which reduced the availability of funds for the support of novel research, and which forced me to approach various cosmetics companies for funds for our sebaceous pheromone research. Of the many to whom I applied, only Proctor & Gamble seemed interested. But it soon transpired that their real interest was rather more concerned with enticing me into working on their antidandruff shampoo. Because of the presumed cytostatic activity of antidandruff agents, they were concerned that their shampoo might run foul of new European regulations on potential carrcinogenesis. So instead of funding my pheromone research, I was asked whether I would study whether (Proctor & Gamble's) dandruff shampoo was indeed cytostatic. I replied that life was too short – and getting shorter. Instead, I offered to review the evidence in the literature and see if I could come up with an independent answer, since from the evidence they presented me with I couldn't believe the story of dandruff as a hyperproliferative disease anyway. That is how, as a commission from Proctor & Gamble in early 1982, I came to review the total published literature on dandruff up until the end of 1981, and from this was able to write a definitive report [1], submitted to Proctor & Gamble in early summer 1982, which finally resolved the problem.

I had found that no single publication had defined the aetiological problem, but that it was possible to proceed by piecing together data from many different sources – a sort of meta-analysis of meanings. Proceeding in this way, I was able to show that there was no clinical and histological distinction between dandruff and mild seborrhoeic dermatitis, and that the underlying causal organism was incontrovertibly the *P. ovale*: thus, all therapeutically effective agents (with the exception of cortisteroids) acted as antifungals by inhibiting this organism; reducing the number of organisms improved the disease and recolonising with the organism led to a recurrence. I therefore concluded that it was impossible not to conclude that dandruff, a mild form of seborrhoeic dermatitis, was the result of an infection with *P. ovale*.

Following this proof, I approached Janssen Pharma UK in the early summer of 1982 and obtained funds to do a study of systemic ketoconazole in dandruff. This study [8] immediately confirmed my predictions that dandruff and seborrhoeic dermatitis were related and would both be controlled by an antipityrosporal drug [2]. It was a short step to demonstrate the curative effect of topical ketoconazole [9] and then to move on to the development of ketoconazole shampoo [10, 11]. There was, Hollywood fashion, a transient block on the road to a happy ending, when it became apparent that what some clinicians considered to be seborrhoeic dermatitis was not responding to ketoconazole. However, it soon became clear that such unresponsive conditions were of a different disease type – mostly flexural eczemas and the like; true classical seborrhoeic dermatitis virtually always responded to antipityrosporal therapy [5]. Now that an effective therapy was available, making a correct diagnosis of seborrhoeic dermatitis had once again become therapeutically important. As in other areas, the advent of a new therapy had resolved nosological uncertainties.

The seborrhoeic dermatitis/dandruff nut was finally cracked; the kernel was *P. ovale*, and the therapeutic squirrel, an appropriate, pityrosporally depressing drug. Ketoconazole was the first drug to be rationally selected, but the principle that led to its use clearly left the field open for further developments, using newer antipityrosporal drugs such as ciclopirox.

9.2
The Development of Ciclopirox Shampoo, the Background

Ciclopirox is a potent, broad-spectrum antifungal and antimicrobial antibiotic, with a reasonable inhibitory profile on various siblings of the pityrosporal family in vitro. Of course, for a variety of reasons, in vitro and in vivo activities do not always correspond; but, nevertheless, the demonstration of antipityrosporal activity in vitro is a prerequisite for testing a drug in vivo. Ciclopirox has long been used in various preparations, including a lotion, cream, gel, and a nail lacquer, and has been shown to be clinically effective against various fungal diseases. But creams are not appropriate to the scalp, and lotions and gels, whilst useable and satisfactory, are often less preferred than a shampoo because of the condition in which they may leave the hair. As with ketoconazole, the obvious vehicle was a shampoo, and studies were therefore done with this product.

First, of course, standard animal and human testing was done to exclude significant toxicity and unwanted reactions. The evidence from studies generated both at Hoechst and at independent laboratories shows the drug to have minimal irritant effect and no contact sensitisation or photo or photoimmune reactivity; the small quantities of drug absorbed from the shampoo are rapidly excreted by the kidney. In addition to the apparent safety of topical ciclopirox, its antipityrosporal potency appears to be related to a unique and novel mechanism of antifungal activity by an effect on fungal cell metabolism without disturbing cell wall and other sterol metabolism, or P450 activity. Thus, the fungicidal and fungistatic effect of ciclopirox seemed worth pursuing in a therapeutic shampoo for seborrhoeic dermatitis and dandruff. Ciclopirox has been noted to have certain effects in anti-inflammatory test systems in vitro and in vivo, but it seems unlikely that this has any relevance to the drug's therapeutic activity in fungal disease.

9.3
Findings with Ciclopirox Shampoo

Many studies have been done, and most have been submitted to drug regulatory authorities, through which they will be available before full eventual publication. As a consultant to this project, I have seen all the data and reports, and my account in this section is based on my reading of them.

A number of uncontrolled clinical studies were done in the course of the shampoo's development. These were part of studies done to ensure a safe kinetic profile and the absence of unwanted toxic reactions, and they showed a beneficial therapeutic effect similar to that seen in subsequent controlled studies. Two major studies were then done in large groups of patients with seborrhoeic dermatitis of the scalp including dandruff; they were randomised, double blind and vehicle controlled. The general procedure was the same in these studies: after diagnostic assessment and a run-in period of 2 weeks, in which only shampoo base was used and baseline severity was established as scale, inflammation and itch, treatment was given in various regimens over a 4-week period, after which the clinical response was assessed; response was assessed again after a 4-week follow-up with a neutral shampoo. The results of these two major studies will be published in full elsewhere, and I will therefore give only a brief summary.

The first study was for dose-finding, using 0.1%, 0.3% and 1% shampoo; the second study was of dose frequency and measured the response to 1% ciclopirox shampoo applied once, twice or three times a week. Improvement was observed in both studies in all the individual components of itch, scale and inflammation and the global score. The response was also apparent from the therapeutic ratio (the ratio of those with a good or very good response to those with little or no response). In the first (dose-response) study, therapeutic efficacy was significantly related to dose, 1% ciclopirox being the most effective compared with shampoo base. From these findings, in the second (dose-frequency) study, the clinical response to use of the 1% shampoo once, twice or three times a week was examined. Therapeutic efficacy was found with all three regimens. From this, a dose regimen of 1% ciclopirox shampoo twice weekly was proposed, and further confirmatory studies are now underway.

Unwanted effects, mostly a tightness of the skin after application, were uncommon; the highest incidence (6%) was in fact found in the vehicle-treated group.

From these results, it is clear that ciclopirox shampoo 1% used once a week provides an effective and safe treatment for seborrhoeic dermatitis of the scalp.

Since this paper was presented in Vancouver, a further large, randomised, double-blind placebo-controlled study, comparing the new 1% ciclopirox shampoo therapy with the established antipityrosporal, 2% ketoconazole shampoo, both given twice a week for 4 weeks, has now been completed; it shows both agents to have a comparable effect.

Of course, since fungal kill by drugs in vivo is always likely to be only partial (the only way to fully demicrobate the scalp is to boil it), recurrences of seborrhoeic dermatitis and dandruff are to be expected, even after treatment with potent drugs. In this respect, the efficacy of ciclopirox shampoo for prophylaxis should become apparent from sensible clinical usage. The results of a further large controlled study of this dose frequency, now almost complete, should add to this evidence. Likewise, further information on the therapeutic efficacy of ciclopirox shampoo in *Pityrosporum orbiculare* infection (pityriasis or tinea versicolor) can be anticipated. Clinical experience will also show the place of ciclopirox shampoo in the often difficult-to-treat patients with AIDS-induced seborrhoeic dermatitis, where existing antipityrosporal drugs may be less effective. It could well be, for example, that ciclopirox alone, or in combination with ketoconazole, which has a different point of pharmacological action, could resolve this often difficult therapeutic problem.

Although, as with any interesting new drug, many studies are still in hand, the results to date are extremely promising and suggest that 1% ciclopirox shampoo will have an important place in the treatment of seborrhoeic dermatitis and dandruff, its minor manifestation.

References

1. Shuster S (1982) Commissioned report to Proctor & Gamble on aetiology of dandruff (and relationships to seborrhoeic dermatitis) and the mode of action of therapeutic agents
2. Shuster S (1984) The aetiology of dandruff and mode of action of therapeutic agents. Br J Dermatol 111:235–242
3. Rivolta S (1873) Parassiti Vegetali, 1st edn. Giulio Spaeroni, Torino, pp 469–471
4. Malassez L (1874) Note sur le champignon de pityriasis simple. Arch Physiol 1:451
5. Shuster S, Blatchford N (1988) Seborrhoeic dermatitis and dandruff – a fungal disease. (Congress & Symposium Series, vol 132) Royal Soc Med, London
6. Shuster S, Thody AJ (1974) The control and measurement of sebum secretion. J Invest Dermatol 62:172–190
7. Thody AJ, Shuster S (1989) Control and function of sebaceous glands. Physiol Rev 69:383–415
8. Ford GP, Farr PM, Ive FA, Shuster S (1984) The response of seborrhoeic dermatitis to ketoconazole. Br J Dermatol 111:603–607
9. Farr PM, Shuster S (1984) Treatment of seborrhoeic dermatitis with topical ketoconazole. Lancet ii:1271–1272
10. Green CA, Farr PM, Shuster S (1987) Treatment of seborrhoeic dermatitis with ketoconazole II. Response of seborrhoeic dermatitis of face, scalp and trunk to topical ketoconazole. Br J Dermatol 116:217–221
11. Carr MM, Pryce D, Ive PA (1986) Treatment of seborrhoeic dermatitis I. Response of seborrhoeic dermatitis of the scalp to topical ketoconazole. Br J Dermatol 116:213–216

CHAPTER 10

Epidemiology of Mycological Infections in Children – in South America

F. M. GONZALEZ OTERO

10.1
Introduction

Mycoses are chronic infections that are widespread throughout the world. They are caused by various species of fungi and actinomycetes that are most commonly found in tropical countries. Mycoses are commonly observed during pediatric dermatology consultations, and their frequency varies according to the geographical area and population [1]. South America extends from 320 latitude North to 550 latitude South; its surface area exceeds 20 million km^2, and it has a population of over 350 million [2]. Within this area, average annual temperatures vary greatly from region to region depending on local factors such as altitude, humidity, and rain. This results in considerable climatic variety. Almost three-quarters of the total area is situated between the tropics.

Fungi exist throughout the world, but there are some species that are specific to Latin America. In our Pediatric Dermatology Section at the Hospital Universitario de Caracas in Venezuela, we evaluated 388 patients affected by mycoses. This represents 3.65% of all patients evaluated between 1989 and 1994 [3], their ages ranging from 0 to 12. Superficial mycoses were the most common (97%), 80% of them being caused by dermatophytes. Of the patients evaluated, 56% were male and 44% female. Although the distribution of dermatophytes was uniform, the largest group of mycosis sufferers (80%) was made up of preschool children and schoolchildren.

10.2
Superficial Mycoses

Tineas are the superficial mycoses most commonly found in Latin America, with tinea capitis and tinea corporis being the most frequently observed. Tinea capitis is present everywhere, although its frequency and etiology vary. For many years there has been a tendency to believe that *Microsporum canis* is the main pathogen, followed by *Trichophyton tonsurans* [4]; we made the same observation, and we also reported a few cases caused by *Trichophyton mentagrophytes* and *Microsporum gypseum* [5].

Tinea nigra is seen in the temperate ecosystems that extend all along the Pacific coast up to Guayaquil and the Atlantic coast as far as Mar de la Plata. The universal cause is *E. wernecki*, with *Cl. castellanii* being the prime pathogen in Venezuela [2].

Tinea imbricata ("chimberé" in Brazil) is the only aboriginal type, and it remains endemic in the Brazilian Amazon, up to the mountains of Lake Atlitán in Guatemala and on the high tablelands of Mexico [6].

Favus, which is caused by *Trichophyton schoenleini*, has practically disappeared. The endemic *Microsporum audouinii* in Santo Domingo is also dying out. Piedras, which are relatively endemic to Latin America, are not commonly observed during infancy and were not detected in our Pediatric Dermatology Section.

10.3
Subcutaneous Mycoses

Sporotrichosis is probably the most frequently occurring subcutaneous mycosis in Latin America. All cool, humid regions, from Uruguay up to Mexico, demonstrate variable degrees of endemic sporotrichosis. The practice of agriculture, the manipulation of the soil and the widespread lack of hygiene, especially in children, make people more vulnerable to the *Sporothrix schenckii* [7, 8]. In our study, we had 11 patients with sporotrichosis of the local and 1 of the lymphangitical kind (Fig. 10.1).

Chromomycosis can be found throughout Latin America and rarely appears in children. *Fonsecaea pedrosoi* prevails in the areas of the torrid zone with more than 600–800 mm annual rainfall, and it is not found in dry areas [8, 9].

Cladosporium carrioni is found in dry and tropical areas with annual rainfall levels of 400–800 mm. The natural habitat of *Cl. carrioni* is thorny flora. In areas where thorny flora grow (e.g., certain sparsely populated states of Venezuela), traumatism by infected thorns is frequent.

The prevalence of fungal infections in the tropical and subtropical areas of the Americas is 10 times higher than in similar areas of Asia, Africa or the Pacific region.

Lobomycosis is an illness specific to Latin America and is caused by *Lobomyces*. It is found in patients living in the neotropical forest, especially the Amazon; in areas where annual average temperatures reach 240 C and annual rainfall exceeds 2000 mm. It is not very common among infants, and not a single case involving children has been published in Venezuela [2, 10].

Mycetomas are not very common in childhood either, and frequently occur in rural areas (Fig. 10.2). The pathogens live in garbage as well as in vegetables. Patients get infected by direct contact through wounds or trauma. In Latin America, the most habitual agent is *Nocardia brasiliensis*, which produces pimples and is found in tropical and subtropical areas.

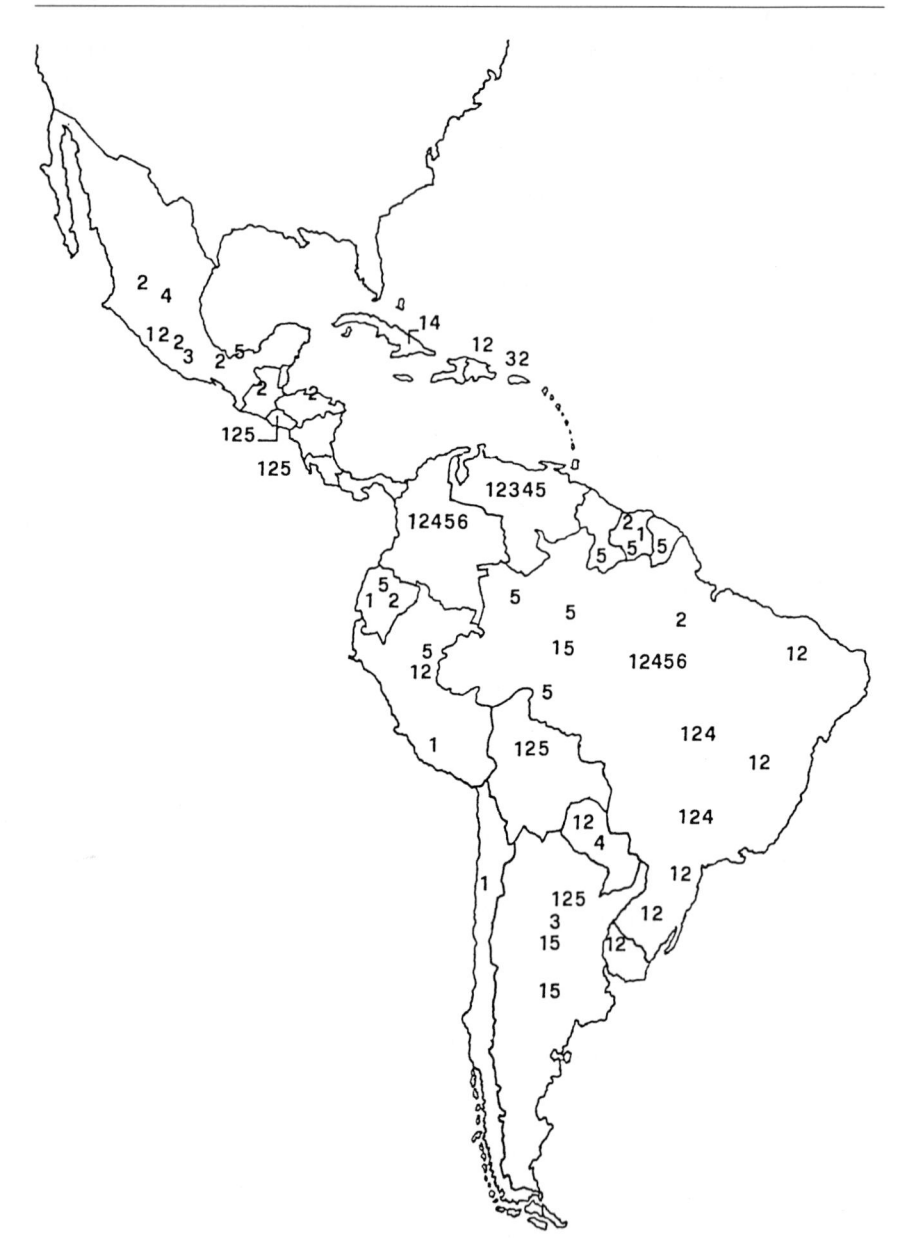

Fig. 10.1. Distribution of subcutaneous mycoses. *1*, Sporotrichosis; *2*, chromomycosis due to *Fonsecaea pedrosoi*; *3*, chromomycosis due to *Cladosporium carrionii*; *4*, rhinosporidiosis; *5*, lobomycosis; *6*, entomophthoromycosis. See Fig. 10.2 for mycetomas

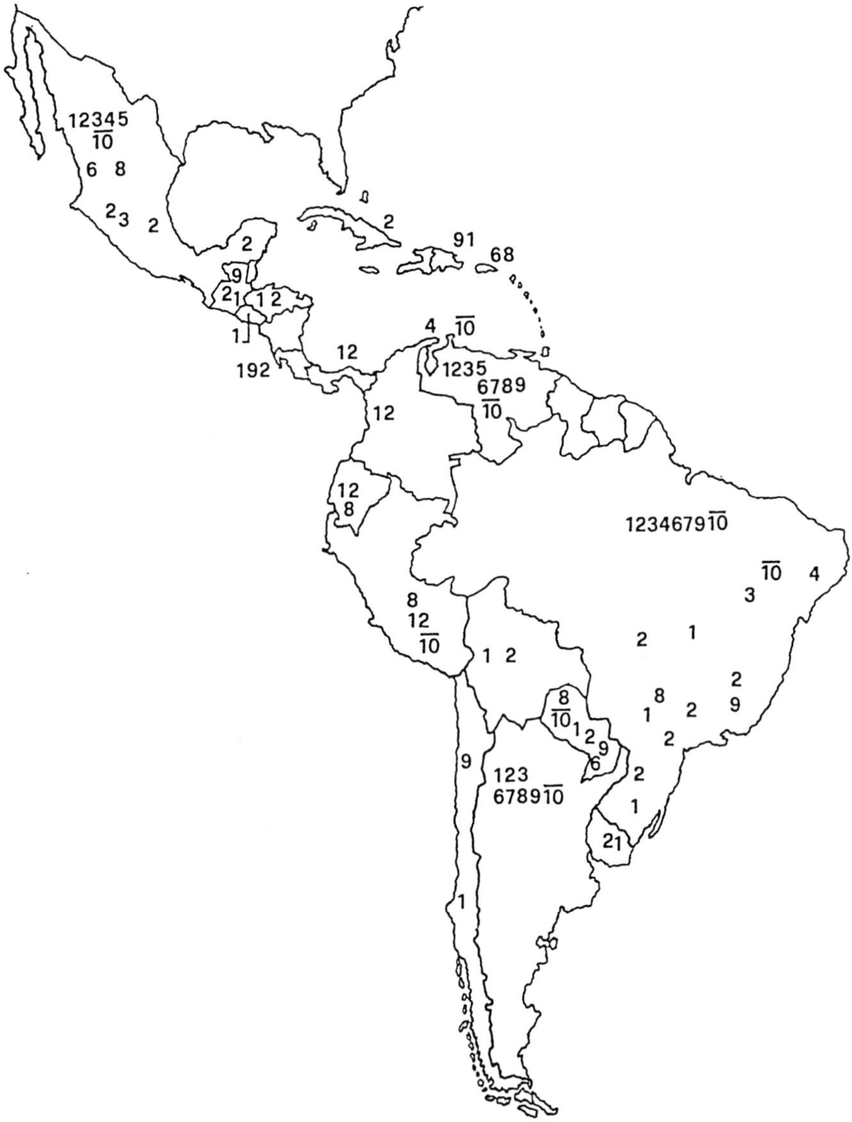

Fig. 10.2. Distribution of principal mycetomas. *1*, Actinomycosis; *2*, *Nocardia* spp.; *3*, *Actionomyces pelletieri*; *5*, *Streptomyces somaliensis*; *6*, *Fusarium falciforme*; *7*, *Acremonium recifel*; *8*, *Scedosporium apiospermum*; *9*, *Madurella grisea*; *10*, *Madurella mycetomatis*

10.4 Systemic Mycoses

Paracoccidioidomycosis is the main systemic mycosis in South America. The incidence rate in endemic areas is 4 cases per million, and 15% of these are patients below the age of 10 years. The causal agent is *Paracoccidioides brasi-*

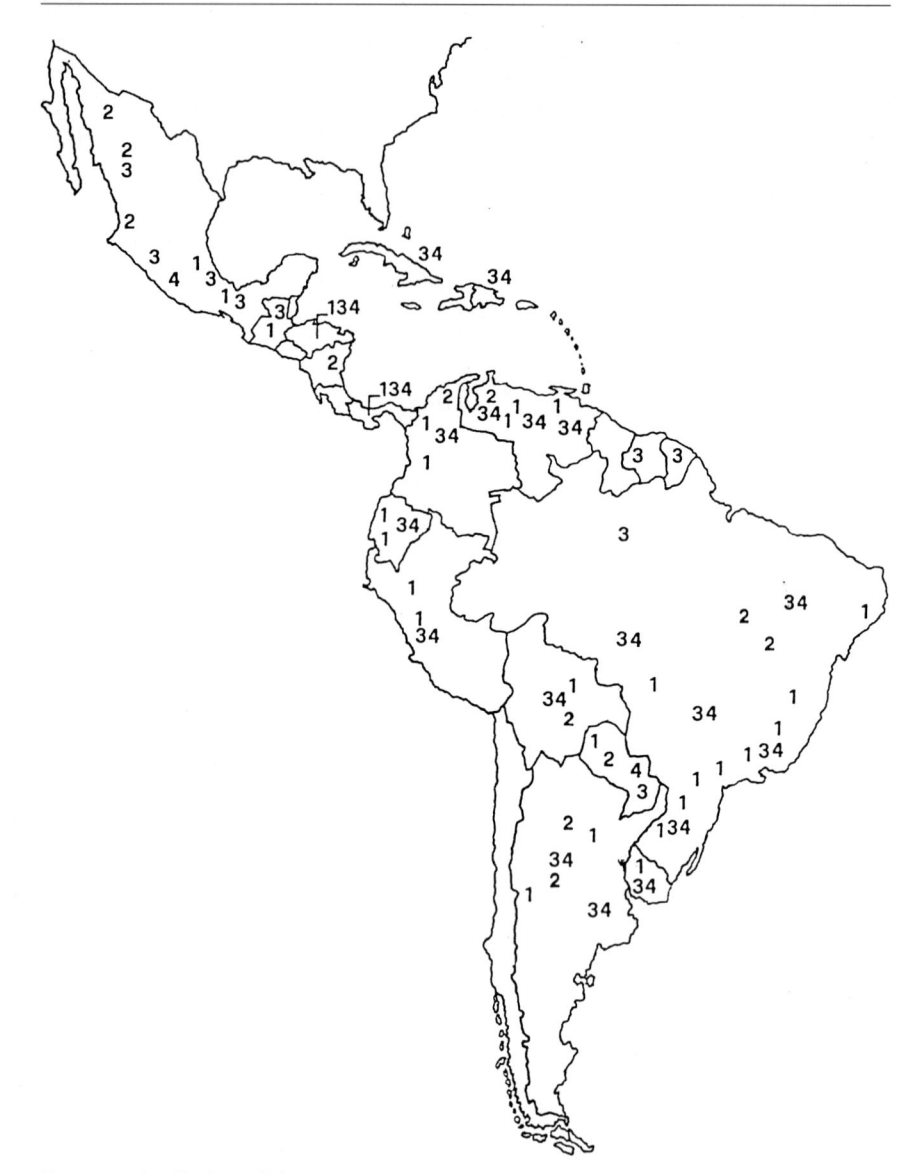

Fig. 10.3. Distribution of deep systemic mycoses. *1*, Paracoccidioidomycosis; *2*, coccidioidomycosis; *3*, histoplasmosis; *4*, cryptococcosis

liensis, which is present in areas with average annual temperatures of 200 C and annual rainfall of 500–800 mm (Fig. 10.3). There is considerable evidence to suggest that 50% of those living in endemic zones might be infected. In our clinic, we had a patient with the disseminated form of the illness.

Coccidioidomycosis is an illness endemic to Latin America, with countless natural habitats in North, Central and South America. These habitats extend from California as far as the pampas of Argentina. The causal agent is *Coccidioides immitis*, which is found in dry areas with less than 800 mm of annual rainfall. The infection is acquired by inhaling arthrospores, which are present in the soil and subsequently transported by the wind. In Venezuela, Colombia, Argentina, Bolivia and Paraguay there are places where as much as 50% of the inhabitants is infected, although disease-related mortality is far lower.

Histoplasmosis, caused by Histoplasma capsulatum, has its largest endemic area in North America, but endemic pockets occur throughout Latin America. *Histoplasma capsulatum* is a saprophytic fungus whose natural habitat is bat-caves rich in guano. Spores are also found in the soil and in the excreta of birds and poultry. Primary infection is infrequent, and the most frequently diagnosed forms are the underdeveloped and the disseminated form [11].

In conclusion, I have attempted to provide an overview of the various types of superficial, subcutaneous and systemic mycosis specific to Latin America and their respective pathogens, and to point out that children are affected by them to a considerable degree.

References

1. Stein D (1988) Fungal, protozoa, and helminth infections. In: Schachner L, Hansen R (eds) Pediatric dermatology. Churchill Livingstone, New York, pp 507–526
2. Borelli D: Mycoses in Latin America. Quaderni di Cooperazione Sanitaria – Health Cooperation Papers
3. Gonzalez F, Rodriguez H. Ruiz A (to be published) Micosis en Niños, en la Consulta de Dermatologia Pediatrica del Hospital Universitario de Caracas. Rev Venez. Dermatol
4. Borelli D (1972) Le Micosi DellAmerica Latina. Bolletino dell'Istituto Dermatologico S. Gallicano
5. Gonzalez F, Rodriguez H, Ruiz A (1994) Micosis superficiales. In: Atlas Dermatologico N0 2. Venezuela
6. Ajello L (1974) Natural history of the dermatophytes and related fungi. Mycopathologia et Mycologia Applicata 53:93–110
7. Lopez Martinez R (1989) Deep mycotic infections. In: Ruiz Maldonado R, Parish L Ch, Beare JM (eds) Textbook of pediatric dermatology. Grune & Stratton, Philadelphia, pp 527–553
8. Borelli D (1969) Reservàreas de algunos agentes de micosis. Medicina Cutanea 4:387–390
9. Albornoz M, et al (1990) Cromomicosis: Reporte de 1 Caso y Revisión de la Literatura. Dermat Venez 28:90–94
10. Borelli D (1961–1962) Lobomicosis experimental. Dermat Venez. 3:72–82
11. Hurwitz S (1981) Skin disorders due to fungi. In: Clinical pediatric dermatology. Saunders, Philadelphia, pp 277–300

CHAPTER 11

Clinical Efficacy of Topical Ciclopirox Nail Lacquer: Double-Blind United States Studies on Onychomycosis

R. Scher

11.1
Introduction

Topical therapy still plays an important role in the treatment of onychomycosis despite the availability of excellent oral drugs. Presented here are the data from the clinical studies of ciclopirox nail lacquer performed in the United States. This preparation has been accepted as safe and effective in the treatment of onychomycosis in many countries outside the United States. It is well known that the disease can be extensive and difficult to treat in many patients, and the response to therapy is very slow no matter what agent is used.

11.2
Methods

Two double-blind vehicle-controlled studies with ciclopirox nail lacquer have been performed in the United States. These multicenter studies were done at nine sites, and approximately 230 patients with onychomycosis were included in each study.

The main entry criteria included clinical and mycological diagnosis of distal subungual onychomycosis of the great toe nail, with an extent of involvement of 25–60%, stratified into 25–40% and 40–60% nail involvement. Age was in the range of 18–70 years, and the patients had to be in good general health. They also met the usual inclusion-exclusion criteria for concomitant medication and medical history.

The efficacy variables were mycology (culture and KOH examination), and the extent of involvement determined by planimetry, an accurate, reliable, and reproducible measurement.

In most previous studies, nail involvement was measured by the distance from the proximal nail fold to the most proximal area of infection (Fig. 11.1). This is not an ideal way to measure nail involvement, and it is preferable to measure the area (Fig. 11.2). To do this, the target nail was photographed (Fig. 11.2a) so that an image of the entire affected area is seen (Fig. 11.2b)

- Previous uni-dimensional method for measurement of nail involvement was inadequate

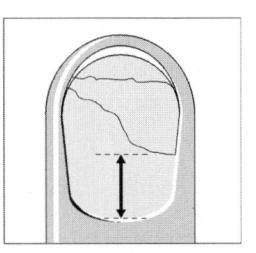

- Needed a way to capture the area two-dimensionally

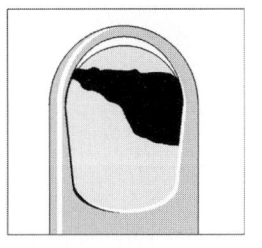

Fig. 11.1. Uni-dimensional and two-dimensional measurement of nail involvement

and converted into a computer image (Fig. 11.2c). The affected area was then measured by this reproducible planimetric method.

The dosing applications for both studies were daily. The treatment period was 48 weeks with a post-treatment follow-up of 12 weeks. The patients returned once every 4 weeks. Photography and mycological evaluations were done at baseline and every 12 weeks thereafter. The patients were randomized in both studies as shown in Fig. 11.3. There were 229 patients in one study and 236 patients in the other, predominantly male over female at about 80% to 20%. The upper stratification numbers with the greater areas of nail involvement were 46% and 38% in the two studies, respectively. The mean age was 50 years (range 18–71) and Caucasian to others in a ratio of 9 to 1. Safety variables were adverse event reports, clinical laboratory results, and changes in physical examination.

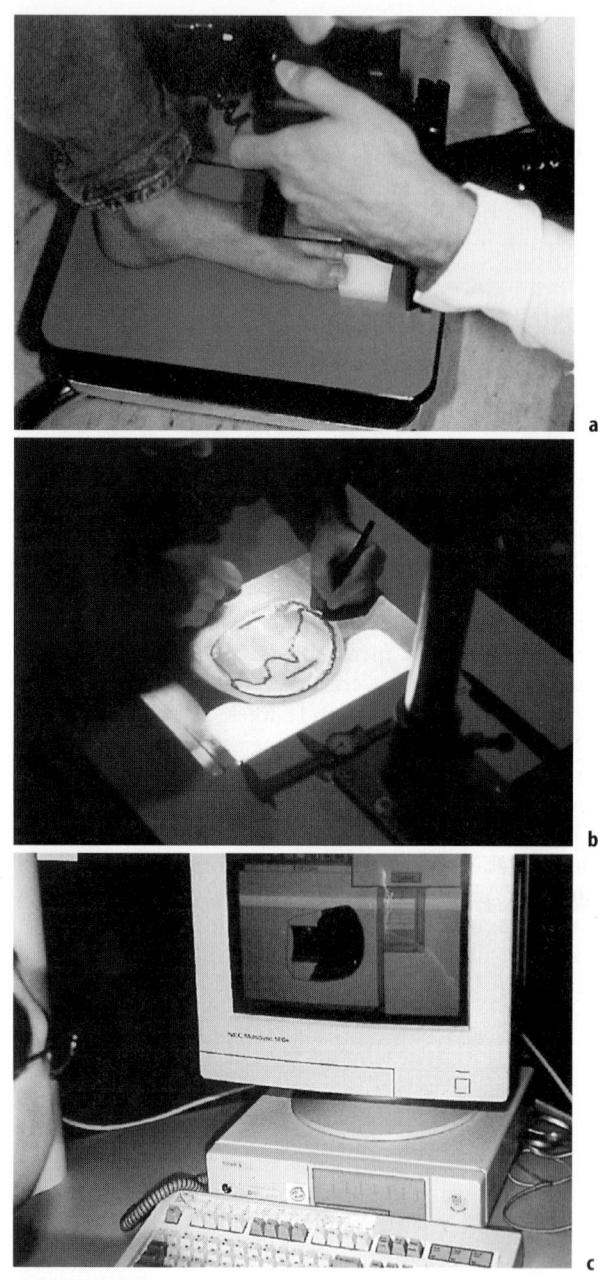

Fig. 11.2 a–c. Planimetric measurement of nail involvement. (**a**) The target nail is photographed, (**b**) an image of the entire affected area is seen, and (**c**) a computer image of the affected nail is created and can be measured

Clinical Efficacy of Topical Ciclopirox Nail Lacquer

		Protocol 312	Protocol 313
▷ Randomized		229	236
▷ Sex	▭ Male	181	182
	▭ Female	48	54
▷ Stratification:			
	▭ Upper (>40%)	~46%	~38%
	▭ Lower (≤40%)	~54%	~62%

Fig. 11.3. Comparison of the patients participating in two double-blind vehicle-controlled studies with ciclopirox nail lacquer 8%

Global Improvement*: Endpoint Per Protocol Analysis [1]

Study	Treatment	Number	Cleared (%)	≥75% Improvement (%)	≥50% Improvement (%)
312	Ciclopirox	106	5.7	15.1	22.6
	Vehicle	103	1.0	2.0	10.7
313	Ciclopirox	114	8.8	17.5	20.2
	Vehicle	112	0	2.7	8.9

* Global improvement was assessed visually by comparing evaluations at each post-Baseline and follow-up visit to the Day 1 evaluation as described below.

[1] The endpoint is the last post-Baseline visit for any patient.

0 = Cleared:	100% clearance of clinical signs of disease corroborated by absence of investigator markings on photograph.
1 = Excellent Improvement:	75% but less than 100% clearance of clinical signs of disease.
2 = Moderate Improvement:	50% to less than 75% clearance of clinical signs of disease.
4 = No Change:	No detectable improvement from Baseline evaluation.
5 = Exacerbation:	Flare of area being studied and/or increase in area of involvement.

Fig. 11.4. Global improvement: end point per protocol analysis

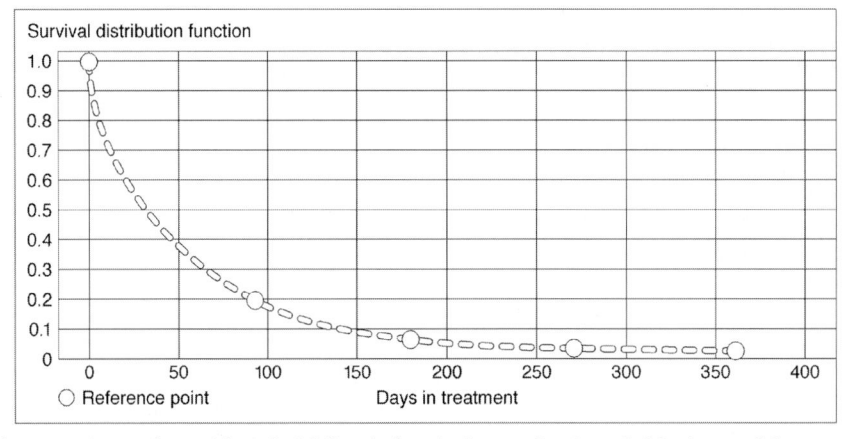

Fig. 11.5. Time to loss of fungal viability (culture) after application of ciclopirox nail lacquer (combined for studies 312 and 313, $n = 200$)

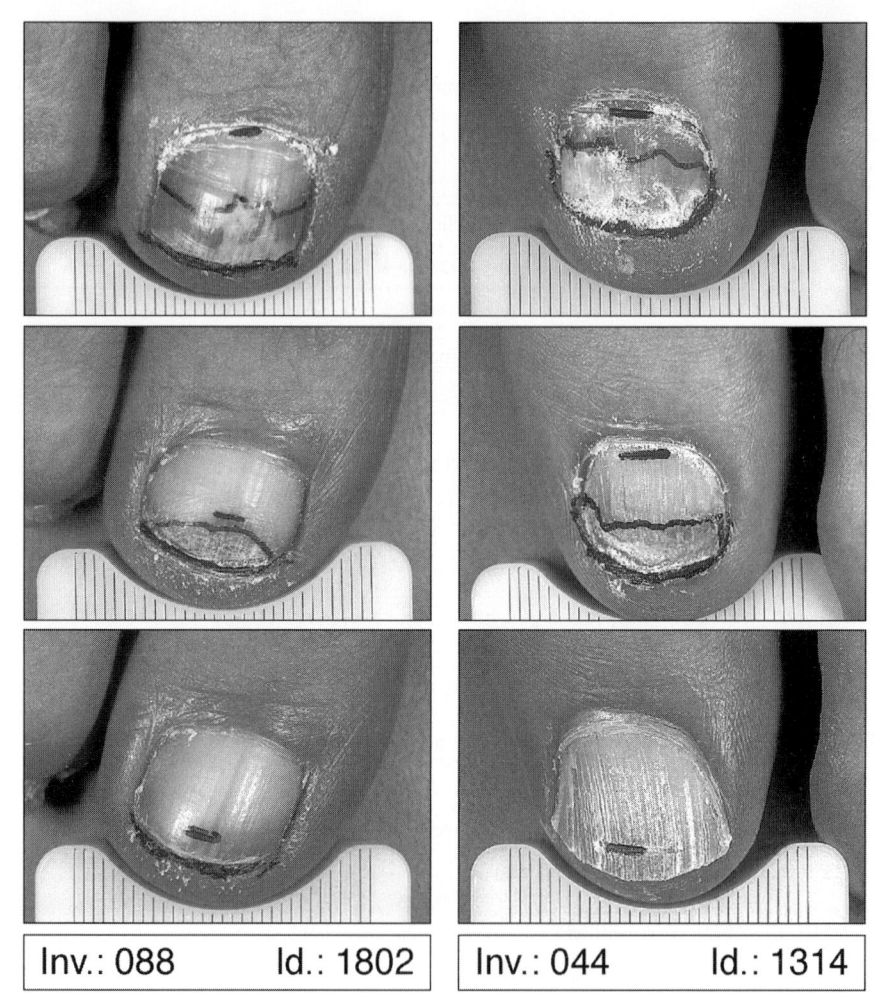

Fig. 11.6. Improvement after treatment with ciclopirox nail lacquer in two patients, demonstrated by photographs of baseline condition and after 24 and 48 weeks of treatment

11.3
Results and Discussion

Clinical success, defined as less than 10% of total nail involvement at the end of the study period, was 15% in one study and 12% in the other. Treatment success, defined as less than 10% involvement with negative mycology was achieved by 13% of the patients in one study and 12% in the other.

The results of the global evaluation are shown in Fig. 11.4. In one study, 5.7% of the patients were cleared, 15% had a greater than 75% improvement, and 22.6% a greater than 50% improvement. This improvement was significantly better than that achieved with vehicle. The observed improvement

Clinical Efficacy of Topical Ciclopirox Nail Lacquer

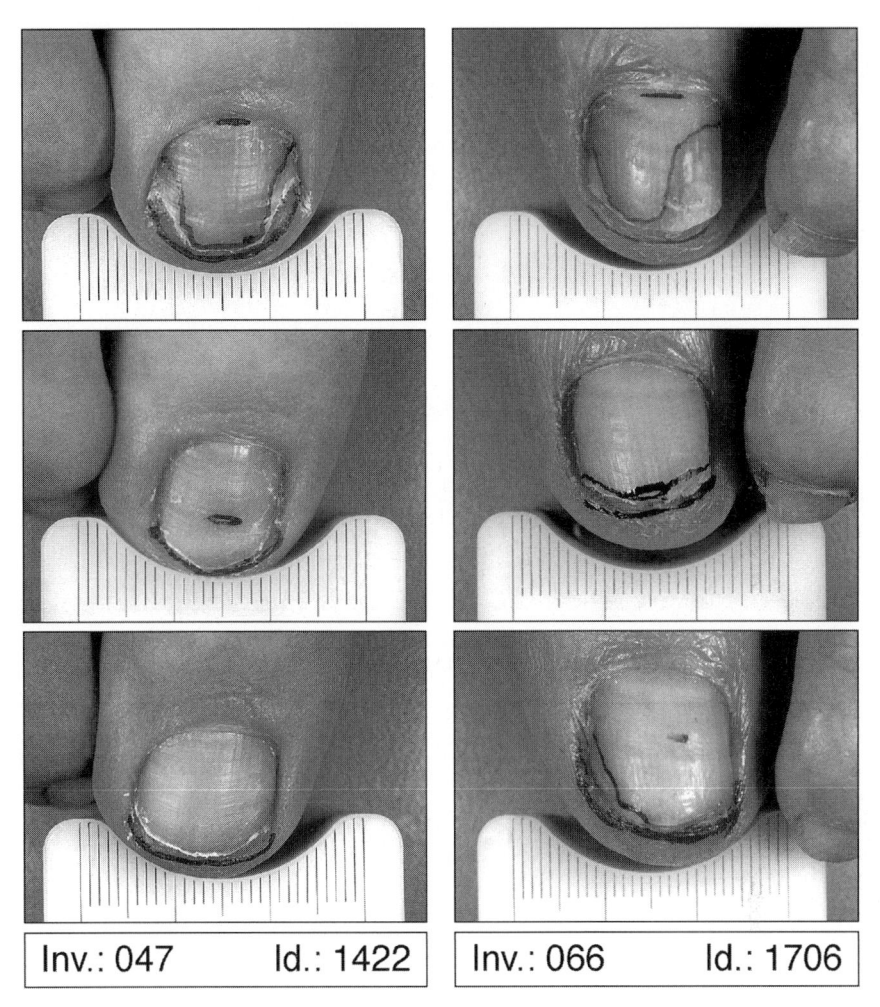

Fig. 11.7. Improvement after treatment with ciclopirox nail lacquer in two further patients, demonstrated by photographs of baseline condition and after 24 and 48 weeks of treatment

with the latter can presumably be explained by the antimicrobial activity of the solvent isopropyl alcohol. The results of the other study were that 8% of the patients were cleared, 17.5% had greater than 75% improvement, and 20% had over 50% improvement.

Fungal viability was also determined, the first measurement being made at 100 days. Figure 11.5 shows a striking decrease in fungal viability for ciclopirox nail lacquer, which increased with time.

Clinical success was clearly demonstrated by photographs (Figs. 11.6, 11.7). The first photographs were of baseline, the next were taken after 24 weeks of treatment, and the last photographs after 48 weeks of treatment. In these photographs, improvement was apparent by 24 weeks of treatment with ciclopirox nail lacquer.

11.4
Conclusion

The goals for treatment in onychomycosis for these clinical trials were mycological cure and 90–100% clearance of the nail plate disease, and this was achieved in many cases. Moreover, the nail lacquer was simple to apply and very well tolerated.

CHAPTER 12

Dose Regimen Studies with Ciclopirox Nail Lacquer

G. WOZEL

12.1
Introduction

Ciclopirox is a broad-spectrum antifungal agent with antiphlogistic properties [6, 8]. Chemically, it belongs to the hydroxy-pyridone derivatives [7]. Clinical and in vitro studies have shown that ciclopirox and ciclopiroxolamine are effective in treating mycoses of both the skin and the nails [3–5, 8, 9]. Much interest has been focused on the development of special topical formulations for the treatment of affected nails. Experimental studies have elicited that ciclopirox easily penetrates into and through human nails [1, 2]. Ciclopirox 8% nail lacquer has been proven to be effective in the therapy of onychomycosis [8]. The aim of the present investigation was to determine the optimum frequency of application of ciclopirox 8% nail lacquer in patients with onychomycosis.

12.2
Materials and Methods

The clinical trial was designed as a multicenter, open, uncontrolled, phase III study, with patients suffering from onychomycosis on both hands and feet. The overall study design is demonstrated in Fig. 12.1. Briefly, the total treatment period lasted 6 months, followed by an additional 4-week-period of evaluation (control phase). The following inclusion criteria had to be fulfilled: (1) male and female adult patients with a diagnosed onychomycosis on hands or/and feet. (2) no age restriction, (3) confirmation of diagnosis by microscopy and culture, (4) acceptable other medical conditions – especially long-term therapy – that did not interfere with trial medications or assessments. Correspondingly, there were the following exclusion criteria: (1) pregnancy, (2) patients who had received systemic antifungal therapy during the last 6 months prior to the study, (3) concurrent use of cosmetic nail lacquer, (4) concurrent local antifungal therapy, (5) limited compliance with the protocol requirements.

For assessment of the effectiveness of the antifungal treatment, in every patient two target nails were allocated, and the affected nail areas were measured

Visit	1	2	3	4	5	6	7	8
Month	0	1	2	3	4	5	6	28 days after end of treatment
Treatment phase								
Control phase								
Personal history/Diagnosis	○							
Inclusion criteria	○							
Exclusion criteria	○							
Demographic data	○							
Patient information	○							
Written informed consent	○							
Clinical investigation	○	○	○	○	○	○	○	
Treatment evaluation		○	○	○	○	○	○	○
Follow-up of the study		○	○	○	○	○	○	○
Mycologic control	○							○
Final protocol								○
Adverse events Concomitant therapy/ Concomitant diseases	only occurrence documented							

Fig. 12.1. Overall study design

using planimetry. According to the frequency of application of the nail lacquer, the patients were assigned to five different treatment groups: once weekly, twice weekly, three times weekly, four times or more weekly, variable application (defined as mode of application that did not fit into any of the other groups). Moreover, the study protocol allowed the possibility of removing affected nail portions by lysis (e.g., carbamidum) or by mechanical means (e.g., scissors, files). The study protocol recommended the monthly assessment of the treatment (improvement, no response, worsening). The overall assessment of drug efficacy 28 days after the end of the therapy by the investigator was made according to the following scale: very good, good, moderate, poor.

Prior to starting the trial, an acknowledgement of acceptability by the Ethics Committee as required by the German Drug Law was obtained, and the study was conducted according to the guidelines of the World Medical Association Declaration of Helsinki in its revised version.

12.3
Results

A total of 1222 patients completed the trial. Of those, 520 (43%) were male and 702 (57%) female. Fig. 12.2 shows the age and sex distribution of the subjects. The predominant age was 50–60 years.

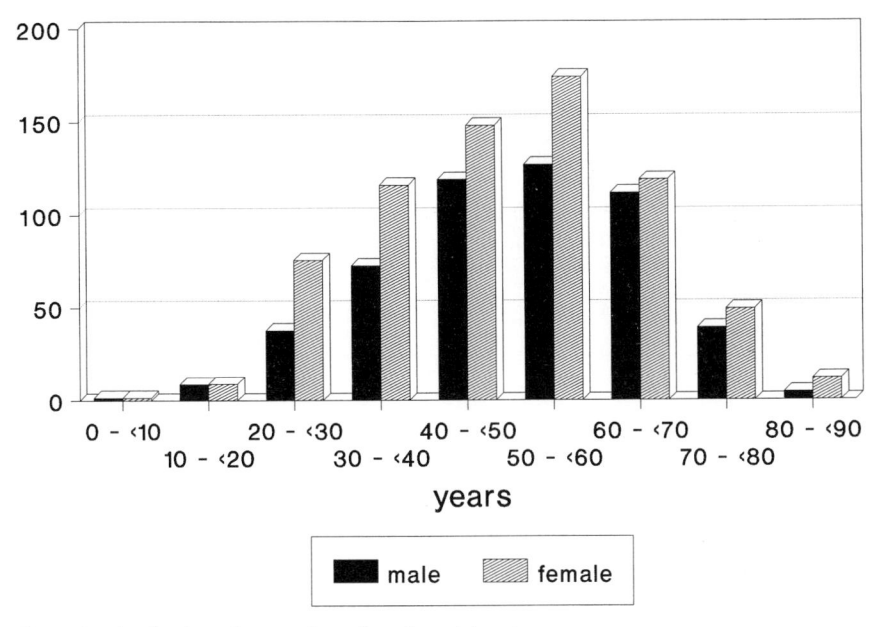

Fig. 12.2. Distribution of age and gender of participants

At the beginning of the trial, mycologic examination by culture was positive in 1013 patients. At the end of the follow-up period, the mycologic control by culture was negative in 883 patients, and the control by direct microscopy was negative in 888 patients, independent of both the treatment frequency and the removal of affected parts of nails. The frequency of infected nails on hands and feet and their respective localization is shown in Table 12.1. The first digit on both hands and feet was most frequently affected. Seventy-five percent of the infections were caused by dermatophytes, of which *Trichophyton rubrum* predominated. Fourteen percent of the infections showed yeasts and – as expected – especially *Candida albicans*. The remaining pathogens were mold (6%) and mixed infections (5%).

According to the recommendations of the study protocol, the investigator, and/or the patients, had to decide on one of the four application frequencies. At the beginning of the treatment period, 20,4% of the patients chose the once-a-week modality, 24,1% twice a week, 25,4% three times a week, and 30,1% more frequently (4–7 times a week). If treated once a week, 51% of all patients showed improved symptoms after the 1st month (Fig. 12.3). More frequent application increased this number to 60 or 63% for twice weekly applications or more, respectively. At the end of the 2nd month, the improvement rate was 59% versus 70% for one or more applications, respectively. However, after 3 months of treatment, these differences all leveled to nearly 70%, independent of treatment frequency. This percentage of treatment success did not change towards the end of the study. Improvement was defined as regression of disease on the two affected target nails as measured by planimetry. In accordance with the study protocol there was the possibility to

Table 12.1. Localization of affected nails

Localization	n	%	
1. Big toe	1646	30.5	82.7% foot
2. Second toe	757	14.0	
3. Third toe	713	13.2	
4. Fourth toe	686	12.7	
5. Little toe	664	12.3	
1. Thumb	279	5.2	17.3% hand
2. Forefinger	212	3.9	
3. Middle finger	193	3.6	
4. Ring finger	137	2.5	
5. Little finger	114	2.4	

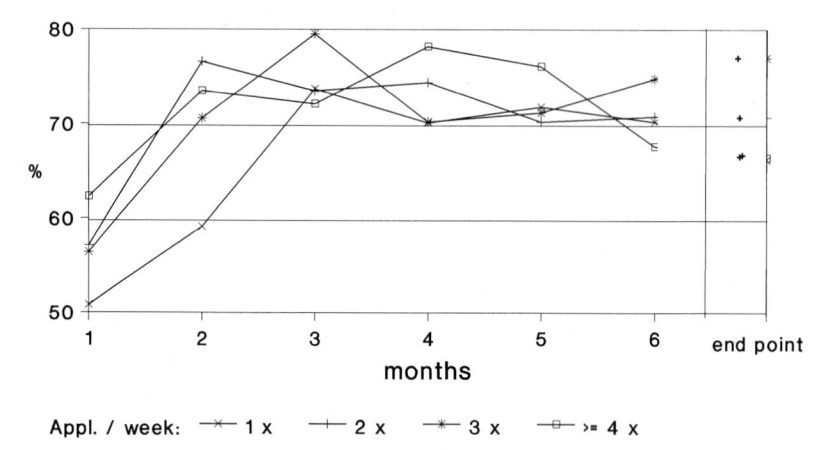

Fig. 12.3. Patients with improved symptoms in dependence of treatment frequency

remove affected nails by non-surgical, partial avulsion by nail lysis (e.g., 40% urea ointment), or by mechanical means at any time of the study. Nearly two-thirds of all subjects had their infected nails removed, whereas one-third remained unmanipulated. It is noteworthy that regardless of whether mechanical removal or lysis were performed or not, the final outcome was nearly the same (Fig. 12.4).

12.4
Discussion

Ciclopirox is a substituted pyridone (6-cyclohexyl-1-hydroxy-4-methyl-2-pyridone) antimicrobial agent with a broad-spectrum of activity against dermatophytes, yeasts, molds, and bacteria [8]. Experimental studies have clearly shown that ciclopirox has the ability to highly penetrate keratinized tissues including human nails [1, 2]. In the nails of healthy volunteers, the concen-

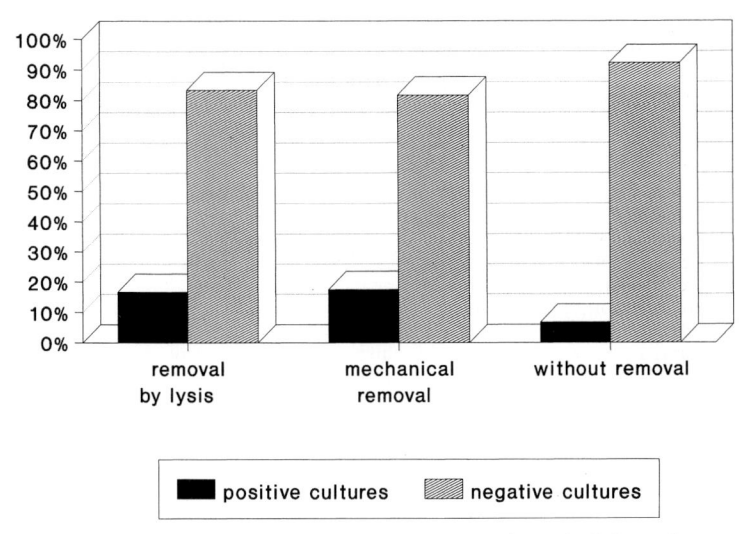

Fig. 12.4. Percentage of positive and negative mycologic cultures at the end of the trial

tration increased during the first 30 days and persisted at a steady state between the 30th and 45th day when ciclopirox nail lacquer was applied daily [1]. The concentration of the compound in the nails were sufficient to kill fungal pathogens [1]. The clinical results obtained in this study reflect the pharmacokinetic and pharmacodynamic properties of ciclopirox. During the first 3 months, the therapeutic response is clearly dependent on the application frequency, whereas after a treatment period of 3 months, no difference in the response to the different dose regimens of ciclopirox application was evident. Accordingly, ciclipirox 8% nail lacquer can be employed for the treatment of onychomycosis in the following sequential treatment schedules. At the beginning of the therapy the formulation should be applied 3 times weekly for a period of 1 month to quickly reach an ungual penetration of ciclopirox and a persistent steady-state concentration. Thereafter, a dose regimen of twice weekly application seems to be sufficient for the next 4 weeks. Up until the 3rd month, the compound should be applied at least once weekly to ensure the antifungal properties. Moreover, the study reveals, that the response rate of ciclopirox at the end of the follow-up period is unrelated to the additional removal of infected nail components by lysis or mechanical means. The therapeutic effect was statistically nearly the same whether patients partially removed affected nail portions or not. Based on this observation, the conclusion can be drawn that patients suffering from nail infections owing to fungal pathogens and applying ciclopirox nail lacquer do not have to remove parts of dystrophic nails. With regard to the compliance, this free choice is clearly advantageous for the patients. In clinical trials to date, ciclopirox lacquer has shown an excellent tolerability [8]. The present study confirmed this. Only in 1.9% (23 patients) of treated subjects were local side effects such as redness and burning (data not shown) recorded.

References

1. Ceschin-Roques CG, Hänel H, Pruja-Bougaret SM, Luc J, Vandermander J, Michel G (1991) Ciclopirox nail lacquer 8%: in vivo penetration into and through nails and in vitro effect on pig skin. Skin Pharmacol 4:89–94
2. Ceschin-Roques CG, Hänel H, Pruja-Bougaret SM, Lagarde J, Vandermander J, Michel G (1991) Ciclopiroxolamine cream 1%: in vitro and in vivo penetration into the stratum corneum. Skin Pharmacol 4:95–99
3. Corte M, Jung K, Linker U, Martini H, Sapp-Boncelet J, Schulz H (1989) Topische Anwendung einer 0,1%igen Ciclopiroxolamin Lösung zur Behandlung der Pityriasis versicolor. Mycoses 32:200–203
4. Frederiksson T, Savopoulos S (1981) Doppelblind-Vergleichsstudie mit Ciclopiroxolamin-Creme und Plazebo-Creme bei Dermatomykosen. Arzneimittelforschung 31:1332–1337
5. Hänel K, Abrams B, Dittmar W, Ehlers G (1988) Bifonazol und Ciclopiroxolamin im Vergleich: in vitro-Studien, Tierversuche und klinische Untersuchungen. Mycoses 31:632–640
6. Iwata K, Jamaguchi H (1981) Studies on the antifungal action of ciclopiroxolamine. Arzneimittelforschung 31:1323–1327
7. Lohaus G, Dittmar W (1981) Zur Chemie von antimikrobiell wirksamen 1-Hydroxy-2-pridonen. Arzneimittelforschung 31:1311–1316
8. Nolting S, Seebacher C (1993) Ciclopiroxolamin. Wegweiser topischer Mykose-Therapie. Universitätsverlag, Jena GmbH, pp 46–109
9. Rollmann O, Johansson S (1987) Hendersonula toruloidea infection: successful response of onychomycosis to nail avulsion and topical ciclopiroxolamine. Acta Derm Venerol 67:506–510

CHAPTER 13

Open Studies of Ciclopirox Nail Lacquer in Onychomycosis – A Review

S. NOLTING

Onychomycoses are disseminated worldwide with a prevalence of 2%–13% or even more in special groups of the population [1-6]. Fungal infections of the nail may occur at any age, but they are very rare in children. They are mainly observed in adults and the number of cases in elderly people is increasing rapidly [7]. Considering the relatively high prevalence and the steadily increasing incidence, onychomycosis should no longer be regarded as a merely cosmetic problem. Onychomycosis may be caused by a variety of fungal agents, including dermatophytes, yeasts and moulds. Infections tend to occur more often in patients with underlying diseases, such as circulatory disorders or diabetes.

Onychomycosis can cause pain from shoes while walking and impairs the function of hands, fingers and feet. Beyond that, onychomycosis can be a social impediment, leading to reduced self-confidence.

Finger- as well as toenails can be infected; however, toenails are much more often affected, accounting for about 73% of all cases reported in clinical studies (Table 13.1) [8-18].

Successful treatment of onychomycosis depends on the stage of infection. In many cases, topical and systemic combination therapy is essential; however, early-stage onychomycosis can often be effectively treated with a topical antifungal alone.

A nail lacquer containing 8% ciclopirox was especially developed for the therapy of onychomycosis. Ciclopirox is a broad-spectrum antifungal agent with fungicidal and sporocidal efficacy, also showing anti-inflammatory activity by inhibiting the formation of 5-HETE, leukotriene B_4, and prostaglandin E_2. Penetration of active drug through the nail plate is a prerequisite for effective therapy. In the case of ciclopirox nail lacquer (8%), this is achieved by the specially developed transungual drug delivery system. After evaporation of the solvent, the ciclopirox concentration in the resulting film on the nail plate is about 35% and serves as a reservoir while the drug penetrates into and through the nail.

Ciclopirox nail lacquer is now available in a number of countries for the treatment of onychomycosis. Successful treatment takes 6–12 months, the duration of treatment being strongly dependent on individual nail growth. Thus, a number of clinical studies using ciclopirox nail lacquer have shown that fingernails require an average 6 months of treatment, and toenails 12 months [8, 9, 11-14, 18, 19]. The efficacy of ciclopirox nail lacquer de-

Table 13.1. Localization of onychomycosis in 1911 patients

Investigator	Patients (n)	Fingernails (%)	Toenails (%)
Effendy and Lüders (1988)	25	13	8.7
Nolting and Lassus (1988)	75	0	100
Xu and Wu (1989)	102	–	–
Adam et al. (1990)	83	0	100
Ehlers and Hübner (1990)	48	11	89
Friederich and Effendy (1990)	58	14	86
Baran et al. (1991)	48	0	100
Effendy (1991)	33	–	
Tai et al. (1991)	100	92	8
Yu et al. (1991)	100	–	
Seebacher et al. (1993)	1239	17	83
Total	1911	27	73

Table 13.2. Mycological cure rates with ciclopirox nail lacquer

Investigator	Patients (n)	Negative culture	Percentage
Ehlers and Hübner	43	32	74
Effendy and Lüders	22	14	64
Nolting and Lassus	75	61	81
Friederich and Effendy	58	49	84
Li Jao Tai	302	282	93
Seebacher et al.	888	748	84
Total	1388	1186	85

monstrated in clinical trials is associated with mycological cure rates of 85%, on average [8, 9, 11, 12, 14, 19] (Table 13.2).

Concerning the frequency of application of ciclopirox nail lacquer, a statistical evaluation by Seebacher et al. [20] in a study of 1239 patients showed that after 3 months of treatment, there were no significant differences between an application frequency of once, twice or four times a week (Fig. 13.1). Thus, a once weekly application is sufficient for maintenance therapy.

In a clinical trial performed by Baran et al. [18], the efficacy and tolerability of ciclopirox nail lacquer was compared with that of oral ketoconazole 200 mg daily in 48 patients who had had onychomycosis for more than 5 years. Patients were treated with either ciclopirox nail lacquer or ketoconazole for 4–6 months. Assessment of efficacy was based on the regrowth of a clear nail plate. At the end of the study, no significant difference in the efficacy of the two groups was found. Ciclopirox nail lacquer was well tolerated in all patients, but side effects occurred in nine of 23 patients treated with ketoconazole, and 4 patients exhibited elevated liver serum enzymes.

According to Gupta et al. [21], adverse drug reactions (ADRs) to systemic antifungals were observed in 10%–20% of patients (Table 13.3). However, hardly any ADRs were observed with ciclopirox nail lacquer, and the overall tolerability was classified as very good or good by 98.7% of the physicians and by 97.5% of the patients [22]. Furthermore, the cosmetic acceptance of

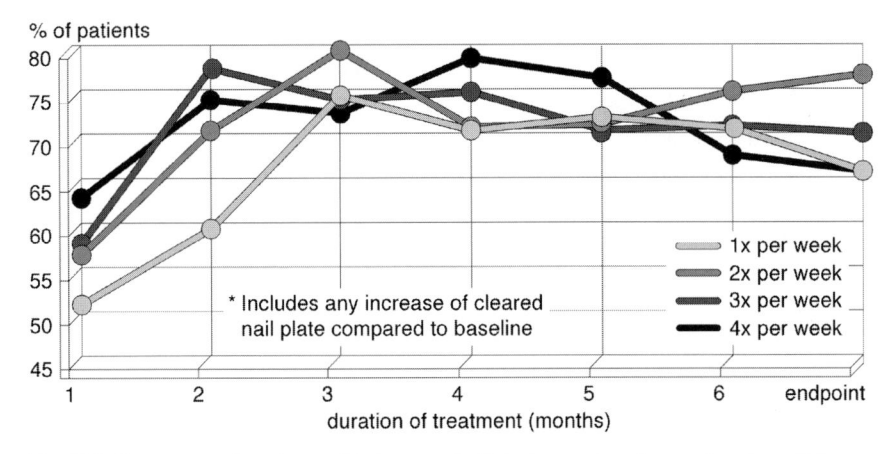

Fig. 13.1. Percentage of patients with improved clinical symptoms* as a function of the application frequency and duration of treatment

Table 13.3. Adverse drug reactions (ADR) (From [21])

Substance	Dosage (mg/day)	ADRs (%)
Griseofulvin	500	12.7
	1000	20.3
Ketoconazole	200	10.7
Fluconazole	150	16.0
Itraconazole	50–200	12.5
Terbinafine	250	10.4
	500	11.0

ciclopirox nail lacquer was high and was classified as very good or good by 85% of the patients [8].

The goal in the treatment of onychomycosis is the eradication of the fungal infection and the regrowth of a clear nail plate. The time necessary to achieve this goal was determined on the one hand by the efficacy of the antifungal agent, and on the other hand by the speed of nail growth. Fingernails grow faster than toenails; however, in the case of onychomycosis, the growth is also influenced by the extent of the nail infection. According to the degree of severity of infection, the formation of new nail plate material is more or less slowed down. Figure 13.2 clearly demonstrates the reduction in nail growth by the extent of damaged nail [23] This has to be taken into account to avoid disappointment and impatience with the therapy. Effendy and Luders [11] found (Fig. 13.3) that if the affected nail area was below 50%, almost all nails recovered after 6 months of treatment. This was not the case, however, if more than 50% of the nail area was affected at the onset of therapy.

In early- or mild-stage onychomycosis, treatment with a topical antifungal agent such as ciclopirox nail lacquer is sufficient. However, in more severe cases, e.g. onychomycosis involving lunula, proximal subungual onychomycosis or total dystrophic onychomycosis, topical treatment has to be combined

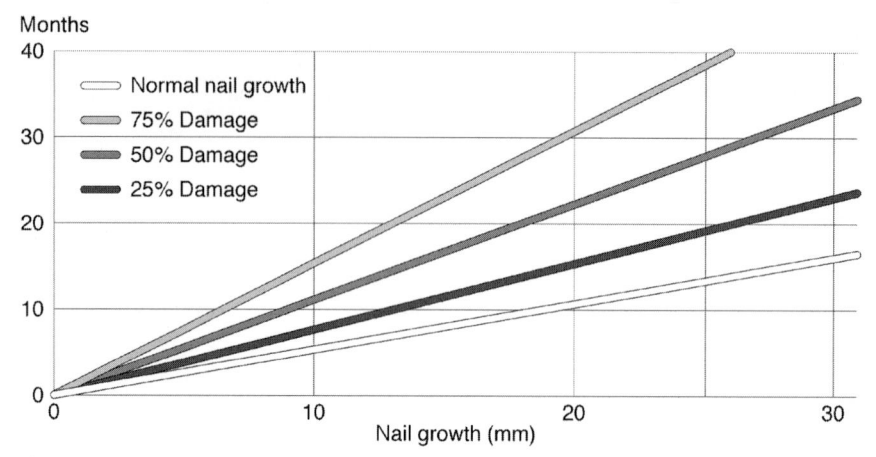

Fig. 13.2. Correlation of the extent of fungal destruction of the nail organ on nail growth

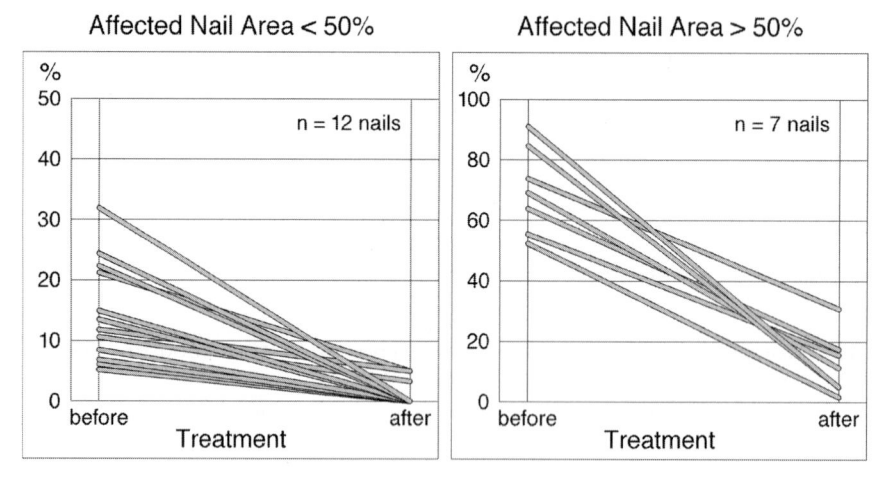

Fig. 13.3. Decrease in the area of the pathologically altered nail plate using ciclopirox nail lacquer

with systemic therapy. After improvement, the systemic antifungal can be discontinued and topical treatment continued as basic therapy.

Recently, an open study of onychomycosis was conducted in our clinic on 117 patients, 66 men and 51 women). Only four patients had onychomycosis of the fingernails, in all others the toenails were affected. The average age was 52.4 years, and the patients had been suffering from onychomycosis from 1 to 20 years (mean 7.6). In 91 patients (77.8%), the infection was caused by *Trichophyton rubrum*, in 12 patients (10.3%) by *Trichophyton mentagrophytes*, in six (5.1%) by *Candida albicans*, and in eight patients (6.8%) the fungi were not identified.

Dosing	
▷ Itraconzole (Pulse):	⇒ 400 mg/daily 1 x week x 3 months
▷ Ciclopirox Nail Lacquer:	⇒ Every second day x 1 month, ⇒ twice weekly for the second month, ⇒ then once weekly until 100% clearance of the nail plate

	Results	
1.	▷ Total therapy success: (= treatment cure + treatment success)	88%
	a. Treatment cure: (= negative mycology + 100% clear nail plate)	41%
	b. Treatment success: (= negative mycology + clear nail regrowing while topical therapy ongoing, time not yet sufficient for 100% clearance due to slow nail growth)	47%
2.	▷ Relapse rate:	12.8% after 2 years without treatment

Fig. 13.4. Topical and systemic combination therapy of severe onychomycosis

The basic therapy used was ciclopirox nail lacquer 8% given during the whole treatment period together with itraconazole, given in a dose of 400 mg once a week for 3 months.

The results of the study demonstrate the considerable therapeutic benefit achieved by this combination therapy (Fig. 13.4). A good therapeutic response occurred in 88% of the patients: 41% of the patients were cured (defined as negative mycology with 100% clearance of the nail plate) and 47% had therapeutic success (defined as negative mycology, with incomplete clearance of the nail at the end of the study. The latter was presumed to be owing to slow nail growth, and topical therapy was therefore continued. After discontinuation of therapy, relapse occurred in 12.8% of the patients within 2 years.

13.1
Summary

Ciclopirox is a highly effective antifungal agent with excellent penetration properties and a unique mode of action. A nail lacquer containing 8% ciclopirox, which was specifically developed for the treatment of onychomycosis, has proved successful in many clinical trials.

Ciclopirox nail lacquer is easily applied and dries quickly; it was found to be highly acceptable by the patients. Cosmetic nail varnishes can be applied on top of the lacquer, apparently without affecting its antimycotic activity. Therapeutic success with mycological cure and regrowth of a clear nail plate was achieved with ciclopirox nail lacquer alone in many patients with mild and early disease and by a combination of the nail lacquer and short-term systemic treatment in severe cases. Besides its efficacy, the nail lacquer was very well tolerated.

References

1. Degreef H (1990) Onychomycosis. Br J Clin Pract 44 [Suppl 71]:91–97
2. Ramesh V et al (1993) Onychomycosis. Int J Dermatol 22:148–152
3. Andre J, Achten G (1987) Onychomycosis. Int J Dermatol 26:481–490
4. Walshe MM et al (1966) Fungi in nails. Br J Dermatol 78:198–207
5. Heikkila H et al (1995) The prevalence of onychomycosis in Finland. Br J Dermatol 133:699–703
6. Gupta A et al (1997) Prevalence and epidemiology of unsuspected onychomycosis in patients visiting dermatologists' offices in Ontario, Canada: a multicenter survey of 2001 patients (poster). Conference of the Am Acad Dermatol, San Francisco
7. Hanecke E (1991) Fungal infections of the nail. SeminDermatol 10:41–53
8. Seebacher C et al (1993) Batrafen Nagellack bei Onychomykosen. Multicenterstudie bei 1239 Patienten. Hautnah Mykologie 3:80–84
9. Friederich HC, Effendy I (1990) Zur Behandlung von Onychomykosen mit Nagel Batrafen (internal clinical report)
10. Effendy I (1991) Stellenwert einer antimykotischen Lokalbehandlung bei Onychomykosen. Hautnah Derm 2:72–84
11. Effendy I, Luders R (1998) Erfolgreiche Onychomykose-Therapie mit Nagel Batrafen (internal clinical report)
12. Nolting S, Lassus A (1988) Wirksamkeit und Verträglichkeit von Ciclopirox-Lackzubereitung (8%) – Nagel Batrafen – bei der Behandlung von Onychomykosen (internal clinical report)
13. Adam W et al (1990) Verschiedene Lackgrundlagen mit 8%igem Ciclopirox. Vergleich der Wirksamkeit und Verträglichkeit (internal clinical report)
14. Ehlers G, Hubner K (1990) Wirksamkeit und Verträglichkeit von Ciclopirox (8%) in einer Lackzubereitung (internal clinical report)
15. Tai LJ (1991) Traitement de 302 onychomycoses. Efficacite d'un vernis a ongle de ciclopirox a 8% en ouvert (internal clinical report)
16. Xu WY, Wu S (1989) Clinical experience with 8% ciclopirox nail lacquer in the treatment of onychomycoses (internal clinical report)
17. Yu B et al (1991) A clinical and laboratory study of ciclopirox nail lacquer (8%) in the treatment of onychomycoses. Chin Med Sci J 6:166–168
18. Baran R et al (1991) Effect of a 8% ciclopirox antifungal lacquer in onychomycosis: a multicenter, double-blind clinical trial versus systemic ketoconazole (abstract 182). 2nd Congress European Academy of Dermatology and Venerology (EADV). Athens, Oct 10–13
19. Tai LJ, Wu S, Yu B (1991) Internal clinical study report
20. Seebacher C, Leonhardt H-G, Horn W (1993) Ciclopirox nail varnish for onychomycosis (internal clinical biometric report)
21. Gupta AK, Sander DN, Shear NS (1994) Antifungal agents: an overview. Part 11. J Am Acad Dermatol 30:911–933
22. Seebacher C (1993) Onychomyleosen – eine therapeutische Herausforderung für Arzt und Patient. Fortschr Med 111 [Suppl 139]:7–8
23. Nolting S, Seebacher C (1993) Ciclopirox olamin: Wegweiser topischer Mykose-Therapie. Universitätsverlag Jena GmbH, Jena, p 61

CHAPTER 14

Influence of Onychomycosis on the Quality of Life

A. STARY, S. TORMA and P.G. SATOR

14.1
Introduction

Onychomycosis of the finger- and toenails affects about 5–10% of the general population and more than 1% of patients attending dermatological departments [1]. The frequency of fungal nail infections observed in medical practise is increasing owing to an increase in the size of older population group, an expanding number of immunocompromized patients, a higher degree of health awareness, and a change in leisure-time activities.

The presence of onychomycosis does not usually lead to severe health problems and therefore is often regarded as a cosmetic rather than a health problem, with the questionable importance of being cured by expensive antimycotic drugs. However, nails serve several important functions: they enhance fine touch and improve tactile sensitivity, aid in picking up small objects, protect the finger- and toetips, may be used as both offensive and defensive weapons, and are excellent tools for scratching [2]. In addition, they play an important role as an organ of communication throughout life and greatly affect the individual's body image and self-esteem. The fungal destruction of nails consequently leads to an impairment of the mechanical functions and may also influence the psychological situation of the affected individual.

Few studies have demonstrated that patients with onychomycosis suffer not only from pain but also from reduced self-esteem and self-confidence, discomfort and frustration [2–4].

The aim of this study was to investigate the impact of onychomycosis on the physical and psychosocial condition of patients with infected toe- and/or fingernails, in their private life as well as at their workplace, by evaluating pain owing to nail destruction; problems in wearing shoes, with grasping of small objects; the attempt to hide nails; the fear of injuries or of damaging clothes owing to affected nails; and the fear of infecting other persons.

14.2
Patients and Methods

14.2.1
Study Population

A total of 1441 patients with nail disorders of the finger- and/or toenails attended the Outpatients' Center for Fungal Infections in Vienna between March and June 1995. Patients were examined for fungal diagnosis and asked to complete an anonymous questionnaire concerning their subjective sense of handicap owing to their nail disorder.

Of the 1441 patients, 936 individuals (65.0%) had onychomycosis confirmed by both a positive KOH test and a fungal culture, and had completed a questionnaire. They were enrolled for further evaluation.

Of the 936 patients, 55.4% ($n=519$) were women and 44.6% ($n=417$) were men. The average age of the patients was 55 years (range 11–92). Of the patients included, 33% were younger than 50 years and 15% were older than 70 years. Demographic data concerning occupation, leisure activities, and duration of disease are presented in Table 14.1 for all patients as well as for different age groups.

14.2.2
Methods

An anonymous questionnaire was handed out to all patients attending the diagnostic center because of nail problems. The questionnaire was subdivided into three main sections. Demographic data such as year of birth, sex, occupation, and leisure activities were collected in the first part, the second one considered anamnestic data, and in the third part patients were asked about their subjective sense of physical and psychological handicap owing to their nail disorder: problems with nail care, pain, problems in wearing shoes, problems with grasping small objects, cosmetic and physical impairment at work, cosmetic and physical impairment in private life, attempts to hide nails, fear of injuries and of damaging clothes owing to affected nails, and fear of infecting other persons by fungal transmission.

Chi-square tests according to Brandt-Snedecor were used for statistical analysis, and the *p* values attached to them were interpreted in an explorative sense and not as tests of a priori hypotheses.

The clinical examination and collection of fungal material were performed by a medical physician. Material for mycological analysis was collected from the distal margin of the involved nail plate using a scalpel. Mycological evaluation included direct microscopy and culture. For direct examination, KOH (20%) with a special ink ("Superquink blueblack") was used. Culture of the nail clippings was performed on two kinds of Sabouraud's dextrose agar with and without cycloheximide [5]. Identification of dermatophytes occurred according to macroscopic and microscopic characteristics of fungal elements.

Table 14.1. Demographic characteristics

Mean age (years)	Total 55		Age ≤50 years 38.7		Age 51–70 years 59.5		Age >70 years 76.1	
	n (936)	%	n (312)	%	n (482)	%	n (142)	%
Sex								
Female	519	55.4	168	53.8	269	55.8	82	57.7
Male	417	44.6	144	46.2	213	44.2	60	42.3
Occupation								
Worker	74	7.9	44	14.1	29	6.0	1	0.7
Employee	291	31.1	179	57.4	111	23.0	1	0.7
Retired	398	42.6	4	1.3	262	54.4	132	93.0
Household	79	8.4	24	7.7	47	9.8	8	5.6
Various professions	94	10.0	61	19.5	33	6.8	0	0.0
Leisure activities								
Sport with special sport shoes	131	14.0	68	21.8	50	10.4	13	9.2
Sport in connection with water	442	47.2	160	51.2	234	48.5	48	33.8
Manual leisure activities	174	18.6	42	13.5	103	21.4	29	20.4
No declaration	189	20.2	42	13.5	95	19.7	52	36.6
Duration of disease								
≤1 year	195	20.8	85	27.2	85	17.6	25	17.6
1–5 years	320	34.2	116	37.2	167	34.6	37	26.1
>5 years	387	41.3	102	32.7	215	44.7	70	49.3
No declaration	34	3.7	9	2.9	15	3.1	10	7.0

The identification of yeasts was performed by the identification of chlamydospores in the case of *Candida albicans* or by the Api-system (bio Merieux/France) in the case of other *Candida* species [6].

14.3
Results

14.3.1
Demographic and Clinical Aspects

Of the 936 patients enrolled in the study, about half were aged between 50 and 70 years (Table 14.2). The majority of individuals (41.3%) had had the nail infection for more than 5 years, with a statistically significant difference between men and women ($p=0.02$). Toenails only (77.2%) were much more often affected than fingernails only (6.7%) or both (13.6%). Fingernails only were more often infected in women than in men (8.9% vs 4.1%) ($p=0.004$). Of the 190 patients with onychomycosis of the fingernails, the thumb was affected in 42.1% ($n=80$), followed by the middle finger in 26.3% ($n=50$), and the forefinger in 24.2% ($n=46$). Of the 850 individuals with onychomycosis of the toenails, the nail of the big toe was affected in 61.2% ($n=520$), followed by that of the fourth toe in 33.1% ($n=281$). The distribution of onychomycosis on finger- and toenails did not differ significantly between male and female or between younger and older patients. Measuring the extent of the changes on the mostly affected nail, in 57.4% more than half of the nail was affected. Male and female patients showed no difference regarding the extent of onychomycosis. Patients older than 70 years had a larger extent of onychomycosis than younger ones.

14.3.2
Identification of Fungal Species

Identification of fungal species demonstrated dermatophytes in 862 cases (92.2%), followed by yeasts in 68 (7.2%) and molds in six (0.6%) cases. Toenails were infected mainly by dermatophytes (83%), followed by an infection together with either molds or yeasts in 15% of patients, and molds and yeasts in only 1%. In contrast, identification from fingernails showed an infection by yeasts in 57%, dermatophytes in 38%, and a mixed infection of both in 5%. A significant difference ($p=0.013318$) in the number of yeast-infections was observed between women and men (10.6 vs 3.1%).

Influence of Onychomycosis on the Quality of Life

Table 14.2. Physical and psychological impairment owing to onychomycosis: differences between the age-groups

	Total n (936)	%	Age ≤50 years n (312)	%	Age 51–70 years n (482)	%	Age >70 years n (142)	%
Problems with nail care	424	45.3	142	45.5	219	45.4	63	44.4
Pain resulting from onychomycosis	201	21.5	60	19.2	109	22.6	32	22.5
Problems in wearing shoes	271	29.0	77	24.7	157	32.6	37	26.1
Problems with grasping of small objects	77	8.2	20	6.4	36	7.5	21	14.8
Cosmetic impairment/job	96	10.3	47	15.1	43	8.9	6	4.2
Physical impairment/job	38	4.1	16	5.1	20	4.1	2	1.4
Cosmetic impairment/private	624	66.7	225	72.1	325	67.4	74	52.1
Physical impairment/private	195	20.8	60	19.2	104	21.6	31	21.8
Attempt to hide nails	397	42.4	139	44.6	201	41.7	57	40.1
Fear of injuries owing to affected nails	116	12.4	38	12.2	63	13.1	15	10.6
Fear of damaging clothes owing to affected nails	302	32.3	94	30.1	161	33.4	47	33.1
Belief in transmissibility of onychomycosis	421	45.0	153	49.0	229	47.5	39	27.5

14.3.3
Physical and Psychological Impairment

14.3.3.1
Pain

Pain owing to onychomycosis was evaluated for location, duration, and extent of nail disorders in all patients, as well as in different age groups. Of the patients with onychomycosis of the fingernails and toenails, 30.2% and 20.9%, respectively, complained about pain. It was reported more often in female than in male patients (Table 14.3). Evaluating the 201 patients (22.9%) who reported pain, toenails (75.1%) were more often affected than fingernails (9.5%) or both (13.9%). More than 60% of patients with pain had onychomycosis to an extent of more than 50%. Furthermore, pain was present dependent on the duration of nail disorders (18.9% for a duration of up to 1 year, 31.8% from 1 to 5 years, 47.3% for more than 5 years). Among the 201 persons who were irritated by pain, the distribution was similar between the age groups but differed between men (32.3%) and women (67.7%) ($p=0,000009$).

14.3.3.2
Physical Impediment

The main physical impediment was reported in connection with wearing shoes (29% of patients with toenail infection), and was especially connected with the big and the fifth toenail (55.8 and 33.3%, respectively; Table 14.2).

Table 14.3. Physical and psychological impairment owing to onychomycosis: differences between female and male patients

	Total		Female		Male	
	n (936)	%	n (519)	% (55.4)	n (417)	% (44.6)
Problems with nail care	424	45.3	257	49.5	167	40
Pain resulting from onychomycosis	201	21.5	136	26.2	65	15.6
Problems in wearing shoes	271	29.0	199	38.3	72	17.3
Problems with grasping of small objects	77	8.2	46	8.9	31	7.4
Cosmetic impairment/job	96	10.3	61	11.8	35	8.4
Physical impairment/job	38	4.1	25	4.8	13	3.1
Cosmetic impairment/private	624	66.7	376	72.4	248	59.4
Physical impairment/private	195	20.8	141	27.2	54	12.9
Attempt to hide nails	397	42.4	275	53	122	29.3
Fear of injuries owing to affected nails	116	12.4	76	14.6	40	9.6
Fear of damaging clothes owing to affected nails	302	32.3	233	44.9	69	16.5
Belief in transmissibility of onychomycosis	421	45.0	250	48.1	171	41

Problems were more often described by women (41.6%) than by men (17.6%) (p=0,000000/Table 14.3).

Of the patients with onychomycosis of the fingernails, 30.7% had problems with retrieval of small objects, especially when the thumb or the forefinger were affected (36% and 31%). No difference was observed in different age groups.

Problems with nailcare were observed by 45.3% of the patients, depending on the extension of onychomycosis, and were reported more often with toenails than with fingernails (Figs. 14.1, 14.2).

14.3.3.3
Psychosocial Impediment

Psychosocial disturbance owing to onychomycosis was expressed by a high percentage of patients hiding their nail infection (42.4%). Especially during private activities, 66.7% of the patients felt cosmetically embarrassed because of their affected nails. Women tried to hide their nails significantly more often (p=0,000000) than men (53.0% vs 29.3%), especially when both the finger- and toenails were infected.

About half of all patients were afraid of affecting other people. This depended on age: while 46.7% of younger patients thought that onychomycosis was infectious, only 28.1% of patients older than 70 years still feared that

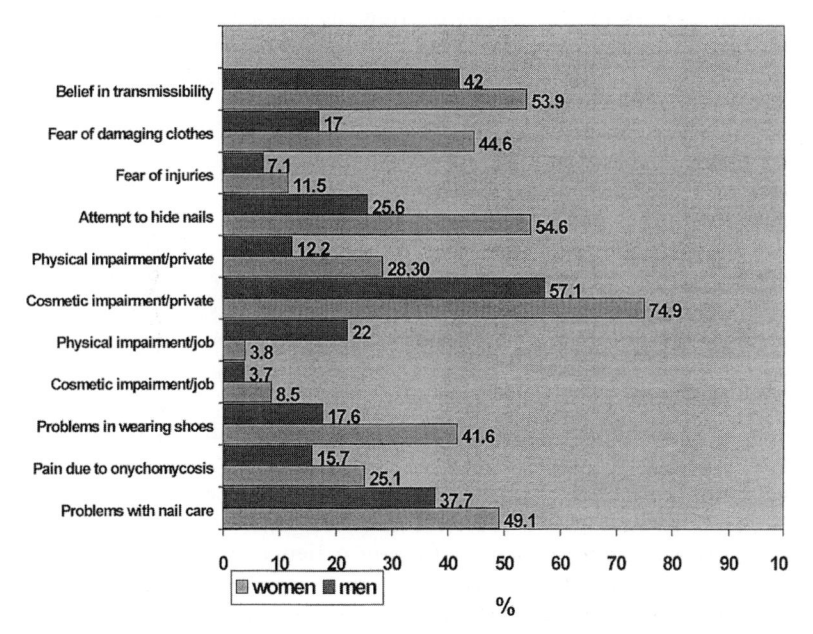

Fig. 14.1. Physical and psychological impairment in men and women with onychomycosis of toenails

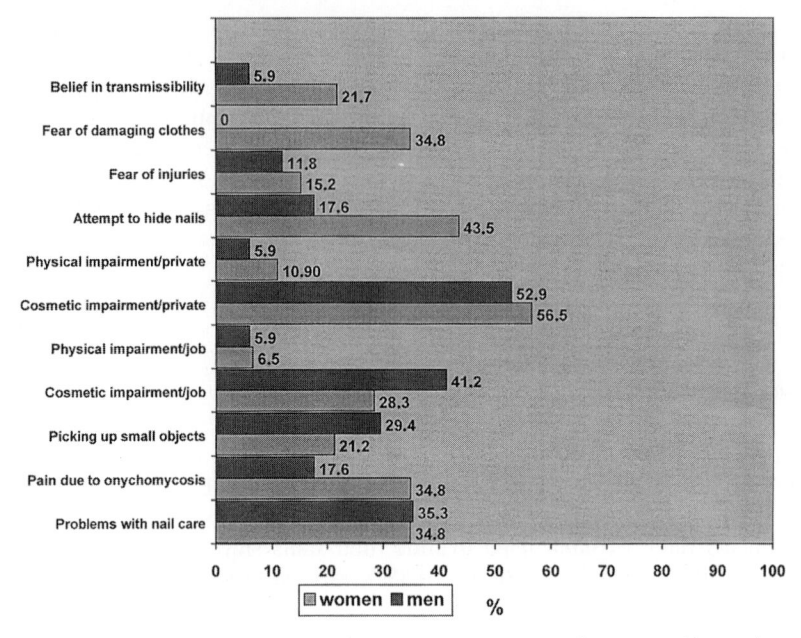

Fig. 14.2. Physical and psychological impairment in men and women with onychomycosis of fingernails

	women	men
Belief in transmissibility	5.9	21.7
Fear of damaging clothes	0	34.8
Fear of injuries	11.8	15.2
Attempt to hide nails	17.6	43.5
Physical impairment/private	5.9	10.90
Cosmetic impairment/private	52.9	56.5
Physical impairment/job	5.9	6.5
Cosmetic impairment/job	41.2	28.3
Picking up small objects	29.4	21.2
Pain due to onychomycosis	17.6	34.8
Problems with nail care	35.3	34.8

they might infect others. Patients were also bothered by the fear of damage to their clothes (32.3%) or of hurting themselves (12.4%). Figures 14.1 and 14.2 give a summary of the results of the evaluation of the questionnaire in men and women differentiated for toe- and fingernails.

14.4 Discussion

Although there has been a dramatic increase in interest in the measurement of health-related quality of life in many medical specialities, few data are available on its influence by dermatological diseases, especially onychomycosis [3, 4, 7]. In a study performed by Lubeck et al. [4], several aspects of overall quality of life (e.g., general health, physical appearance, social functioning and confidence, well-being, bodily pain) among patients with onychomycosis were compared with persons not suffering from onychomycosis. Those with onychomycosis had a significantly reduced quality of life.

The aim of the present study was to investigate physical and psychosocial factors influencing the quality of life in patients with onychomycosis as a basis for further discussion on the necessity of treatment procedures. In the present study, the majority of patients (41.3%) had suffered from onychomycosis for a long time. The visual appearance of the mycologically changed toe- and fingernails in the private life was the main impact on the health condition and was reported by more than 60% of the patients. Although women felt more often embarrassed than men, 25% of the men tried to hide their affected nails. The fear of transmitting the fungal infection to other persons was reported in an unexpectedly high percentage (about 50%) and was more often observed among younger patients. Onychomycosis had a negative impact on everyday activities such as grasping and picking up small objects, by the fear of damaging clothes, and by minor injuries. Furthermore, nail infections had an influence on leisure activities. Owing to longer life expectancy, better health conditions, and increased possibilities of leisure activities, onychomycosis was a handicap not only for younger patients but also for older persons considering sporting and other leisure activities. Pain was reported by a high percentage of women, leading to problems with wearing shoes, especially in patients with a longer duration of onychomycosis of the toenails. Differentiating the physical and psychological impairment between different age-groups, problems with picking up small objects increased with increasing age, while the fear of transmissibility as well as cosmetic impairment decreased with increasing age.

The data are in concordance with those presented earlier, where persons with onychomycosis suffered embarrassment from exposing their nails; they feared intimate situations, and had difficulty with work-related activities requiring the use of the fingers [4]. While patients may adapt to their psychosocial problems, the physical discomfort still remains in a high percentage of patients, especially in those suffering from onychomycosis for a long time. This may lead to a reduced ability to perform leisure activities in the private life, as well as to a handicap during work.

In summary, the data confirm the impact of onychomycosis on the physical and psychosocial health in a large study group suffering from fungal nail changes. This negative influence on the patient's quality of life should encourage physicians to reconsider effective therapeutic measures to cure fungal infections of the nails, even in older patients.

14.5
Summary

Onychomycosis is often regarded as a primarily cosmetic problem and may therefore not necessarily require effective medical treatment. However, the nails serve several important functions, and in consequence of onychomycosis their use is affected adversely.

The aim of this study was to evaluate the impairment of onychomycosis on physical and psychosocial conditions of patients and its influence on the quality of life. Of the 1441 patients with nail disorders, 936 individuals (65.0%) suffered from onychomycosis, diagnosed by a positive KOH test and fungal culture, and completed an anonymous questionnaire about the influence of nail disorders on their profession, leisure activities, and psychological situation.

A high percentage of patients felt disturbed by the fungal nail infection owing to pain (21.5%); physical impediment (at work 4.1%, at leisure

20.8%); psychological problems, especially in private activities (67%); and the fear of transmissibility to other persons (45%). Patients over 70 years of age reported problems similar to younger ones concerning the disturbance of leisure activities.

The results confirm that onychomycosis is not only a cosmetic problem, but may also cause health and psychological disturbances and therefore requires effective therapeutic measures.

Acknowledgements. The authors acknowledge the support of this project by Janssen-Cilag, Austria, and are grateful for special advice in the evaluation of the questionnaire from Bettina Schricker, Janssen-Cilag, Austria.

References

1. Blecher P, Korting HC (1993) A new combined diagnostic approach to clinically and microscopically suspected onychomycosis unproven by culture. Mycosis 36:321–324
2. Scher RK (1994) Onychomycosis is more than a cosmetic problem. Br J Dermatol [Suppl] 43:15
3. Finlay AY, Khan GK (1994) Dermatology Life Quality Index (DLQI) – a simple practical measure for routine clinical use. Clin Exp Dermatol 19:210–216
4. Lubeck DP, Patrick DL, McNulty P, Fifer SK, Birnbaum I (1993) Quality of life of persons with onychomycosis. Qual Life Res 2:341–348
5. McGinnis MR (1980) Laboratory handbook of medical mycology. Academic Press, New York London, pp 576–577
6. McGinnis MR (1980) Laboratory handbook of medical mycology. Academic Press, New York London, pp 352–357
7. Finlay AY, Coles EC (1995) The effect of severe psoriasis on the quality of life of 369 patients. Br J Dermatol 132:236–244

CHAPTER 15

Treatment of Onychomycoses: Pharmacoeconomic Aspects

T. R. EINARSON, P. I. OH and N. SHEAR

15.1
Introduction

Onychomycosis is a condition that affects about 2%–3% of all people [1]. It tends to be chronic, with many recurrences, and thus represents a major health issue. Older antifungal agents have low rates of clinical effectiveness as well as many unacceptable side effects [adverse drug reactions (ADRs)] [2]. Newer oral agents, although more effective, still produce ADRs and are more costly than older preparations; nonetheless, they are more cost effective, despite higher acquisition costs [3].

Topical lacquers have been recently introduced into several countries as an alternative to oral therapies [4, 5]. While their efficacy is somewhat lower than that of oral agents, they are not associated with significant ADRs and their acquisition costs are considerably lower [3]. The purpose of the present study was to determine the pharmacoeconomic status of topical lacquers compared with oral agents when used for treating mild-to-moderate onychomycosis from a government payer perspective.

15.2
Methods

Two topical lacquers, amorolfine (AMO) and ciclopirox (CIC), and the oral agents griseofulvin (GRI), itraconazole (ITR), and terbinafine (TER) were examined for treatment of dermatophyte onychomycosis in Canada, France, Germany, Italy, Spain, the United Kingdom, and the United States. A predictive (decision tree) model was used to compare drugs [6]. Expert panels were assembled to determine clinical practice patterns and reimbursement practices in each country. Meta-analysis [7] was used to determine clinical success rates and relapse rates, and standard costs were used in each country. The perspective was that of the government payer. All direct costs were included, while indirect costs and costs of treating ADRs were not considered. The expected cost per patient treated and the cost per disease-free day were calculated. Data were analyzed over a 5-year horizon, with a 5% discounting rate. The sensitivity of the model was examined using Rank Order Stability Analysis (ROSA) [8].

15.3
Results

A total of 55 studies of at least one of the study drugs in onychomycosis were identified in the literature search. Of those studies, 22 were excluded for the following reasons: lack of data (4), inappropriate patients (1), inappropriate infecting organism (1), inappropriate regimen (4), not clinical trial (9), and duplication (3). Consequently, 33 studies comprising 59 clinical arms that reported data from 3595 patients were used; 27 of those trials presented data from 1387 patients for relapse.

Table 15.1 presents event rates from the meta-analysis. Those probabilities were combined with costs in a decision tree model to derive the expected costs for each drug. The expected cost is the weighted average cost for a typical patient, considering the drug's success rate and treatments used in failures. It incorporates all direct costs, including medical care, drug costs, and laboratory tests. We also calculated the expected cost per symptom-free day (SFD) by using a 5 year time horizon, which allowed adequate time for all patients to be treated, retreated in cases of relapse, or administered an adequate course of back-up treatment in cases of failure. Days when treatment was not required (i.e., SFDs) were summed for each drug, then divided into the expected cost and compared.

Table 15.2 presents the results of the pharmacoeconomic analyses, in local currency. In all countries, ciclopirox had the lowest expected cost and cost per SFD. Figures 15.1 and 15.2 illustrate these results with all costs expressed in US dollars as a standard measurement. Sensitivity analyses or probabilities and costs over relevant ranges showed that the baseline results were robust.

15.4
Discussion

When considering results, it should be noted that there were few randomized controlled trials available, so open trials, often without controls, were used.

Table 15.1. Summary of primary clinical rates for onychomycosis

Drug	Trials	Patients	Cure	Improved	Fail	Relapse
Amorolfine	3	622	0.358	0.289	0.353	0.139
Ciclopirox	11	1719	0.313	0.265	0.422	0.136
Griseofulvin	20	576	0.273	0.396	0.331	0.318
Itraconazole	14	331	0.488	0.391	0.121	0.270
Terbinafine	11	426	0.776	0.123	0.101	0.088

Table 15.2. Expected costs per treated patient for each drug (in US Dollar)

Analysis	Country	Drug				
		AMO	CIC	GRI	ITR	TER
Expected cost	Canada ($CDN)	389	344	1138	690	571
	France (FFr)	1304	1259	3393	4551	2544
	Germany (DM)	418	406	2423	990	735
	Italy (Lire)	386623	370206	1225042	895542	702706
	Spain (Ptas)	66792	57446	149610	92903	73959
	United Kingdom (£)	439	353	748	490	402
	United States (US $)	614	538	2018	1153	735
Cost/Symptom Free Day	Canada ($CDN)	0.25	0.21	0.94	0.42	0.34
	France (FFr)	0.85	0.76	2.82	2.74	1.50
	Germany (DM)	0.27	0.25	2.01	0.60	0.43
	Italy (Lire)	252	224	1017	540	414
	Spain (Ptas)	43.54	34.76	124.21	55.99	43.58
	United Kingdom (£)	0.29	0.21	0.62	0.30	0.24
	United States (US $)	0.45	0.36	1.91	0.77	0.48

AMO, amorolfine; CIC, ciclopirox; GRI, griseofulvin; ITR, itraconazole; TER, terbinafine.

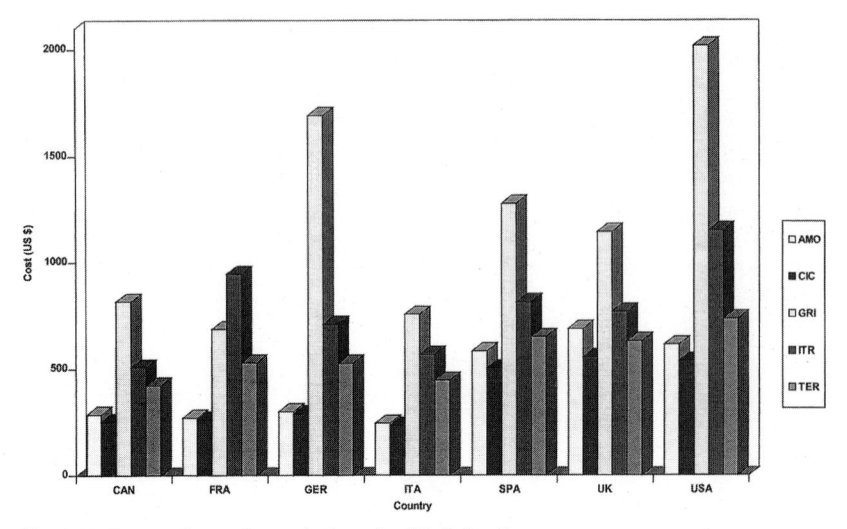

Fig. 15.1. Expected cost for each drug (in US dollars)

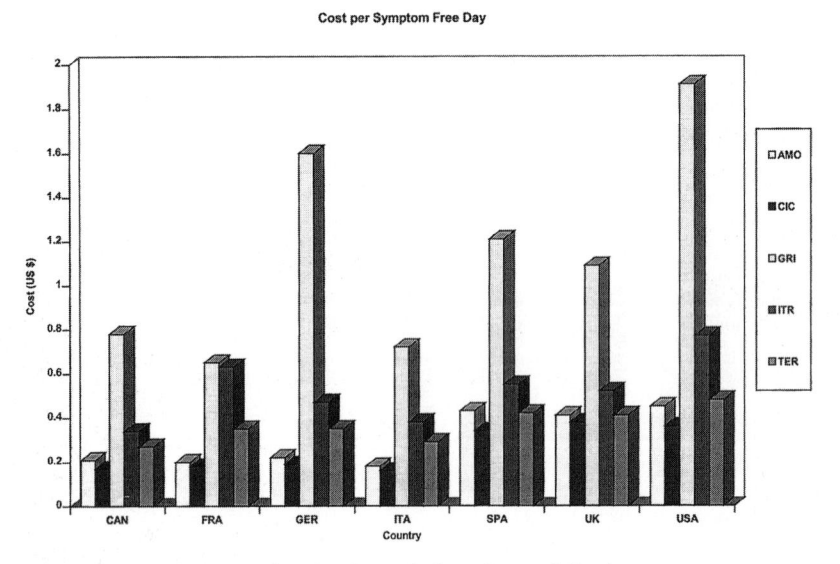

Fig. 15.2. Cost per disease-free day for each drug (in US dollars)

However, the numbers of patients treated were large, and overall rates were comparable to those from randomized trials. Furthermore, data for topical lacquers were derived mainly from patients having mild-to-moderate onychomycoses involving between two and four nails on average, but mainly toenails (80%). On the other hand, data for oral drugs represented a broader range from mild-to-severe involvement of both fingernails and toenails; hence, the results should be interpreted accordingly.

Also of note is the fact that the costs of side effects were excluded from consideration. The topical agents reported very few problems, the majority of which were mainly local irritation, which required no further treatment and seldom (if ever) resulted in a change in treatment. On the other hand, oral agents have produced a number of well documented serious ADRs such as hepatotoxicity, taste disorder, and blood dyscrasias. Therefore, there may have been some bias against the topical preparations.

This analysis was really a comparison of management strategies rather than of single antifungal agents in isolation. For patients with mild onychomycosis (i.e., less than five nails), a non-systemic therapy would intuitively be more acceptable, and given the larger difference in acquisition costs between oral and topical therapies, a strategy employing a lacquer initially with oral as back-up would also be economically attractive. This hypothesis was confirmed by this analysis. Measures of patient preference, such as utilities and quality of life might provide further evidence in this regard and should be explored in further studies.

15.5
Conclusions

We conclude that a management strategy employing CIC nail lacquer as the initial therapy is the most cost-effective regimen for the treatment of mild-to-moderate onychomycosis. These results were consistent in all seven countries examined. Topical therapies provide moderate clinical effectiveness at a reasonable price, while avoiding the side effects produced by oral therapies.

References

1. Roberts DT (1992) Prevalence of dermatophyte onychomycosis in the United Kingdom: results of an omnibus survey. Br J Dermatol 126:23–27
2. Gupta AK, Sauder DN, Shear NH (1994) Continuing medical education: antifungal agents: an overview. J Am Acad Dermatol 30:677–698, 911–933
3. Einarson TR, Gupta A, Shear NH, Arikian SR (1996) Clinical and economic factors in the treatment of onychomycosis. PharmacoEconomics 9:307–320
4. Pittrof F, Gerhards J, Erni W, Klecak G (1992) Loceryl nail lacquer – realization of a new galencial approach to onychomycosis therapy. Clin Exper Dermatol 17:26–28
5. Seebacher C, Ulbricht H, Worz K (1993) Behandlungsergebnisse einer multicenter studie mit Ciclopirox-Nagellack bei onychomykosen. Hautnah Myk 3:80–84
6. Einarson TR, Shear NH, Oh PI (1997) Models for pharmacoeconomic analysis. Can J Clin Pharmacol 4:25–29
7. Einarson TR (1997) Pharmacoeconomic applications of meta-analysis for single groups: antifungal onychomycosis lacquers as example. Clin Ther 19:559–569
8. Einarson TR, Arikian SR, Doyle J (1995) Rank order stability analysis (ROSA): testing pharmacoeconomic data. Med Decis Making 15:367–372

# The Safety Aspects of Systemic and Topical Antifungal Agents Used in the Management of Onychomycosis

A. K. GUPTA

Abstract

When deciding upon the optimal antifungal agent for treating onychomycosis, the safety profile of the available agents is an important consideration. The topical antifungal agents have adverse events that are localized to the application site, and these are generally not as significant as the adverse effects that may occur with oral agents. The drug of choice is the most cost-effective antimycotic with an acceptable adverse-events profile.

16.1 Introduction

There are several properties of antifungal agents that need to be evaluated when considering the best antimycotic to treat onychomycosis. These include the route of drug delivery (topical versus oral), efficacy, dosage schedule, safety issues (including the frequency and spectrum of adverse effects and drug interactions), and cost of therapy. The safety aspects of oral and topical antifungal agents used in the treatment of onychomycosis will be discussed in this review.

16.2 Traditional Antifungal Agents for the Treatment of Onychomycosis

16.2.1 Griseofulvin

In 1958, griseofulvin became the first significant antifungal agent available for the management of dermatomycoses such as tinea capitis; however, it was relatively ineffective in pedal onychomycosis [1]. It had a narrow spectrum, with only dermatophytes responding to griseofulvin therapy; it was ineffective against *Candida* species and non-dermatophyte molds.

Adverse effects with griseofulvin may occur in 10–15% of patients, with the more frequent reactions being nausea, vomiting, epigastric distress, diarrhea, headache, cutaneous eruption, and urticaria; some of these are dose-dependent. Occasionally, fatigue, dizziness, insomnia, mental confusion, and impairment of the performance of routine activities may occur. Rare adverse events include hepatic toxicity, gastrointestinal bleeding, menstrual irregularities and paresthesias of the hands and feet, proteinuria, leukopenia and granulocytopenia. Some of the serious side-effects have occurred at high doses of griseofulvin or with long duration of therapy. Griseofulvin interferes with porphyrin metabolism and may precipitate porphyria attacks. Furthermore, griseofulvin may precipitate or exacerbate lupus erythematosus. Photosensitivity reactions can occur, and the patient should be cautioned about prolonged exposure to sunlight. Griseofulvin is contraindicated in hepatocellular failure.

Drug interactions with griseofulvin include anticoagulants (coumarin- or indandione-derivative) (decrease in hypoprothrombinemic activity of the anticoagulant), barbituates or primidone (decreased griseofulvin levels), contraceptives (decreased contraceptive effectiveness), and alcohol (potentiation of alcohol effects).

With regard to laboratory monitoring, one possible scheme is complete blood count with differential and liver enzymes at pretherapy and thereafter every 2 months; however, the role of monitoring has been questioned [2].

16.2.2
Ketoconazole

Ketoconazole became available for use in the late 1970s. The initial enthusiasm for the use of this first broad-spectrum agent in the treatment of dermatomycoses was tempered by reports of hepatotoxicity (incidence 1:10,000 to 1:15,000 exposed patients), with rare fatalities [3, 4]. In these patients, the median duration of therapy before the development of symptomatic hepatotoxicity was 28 days, although there were instances when the range extended to as low as 3 days. The hepatic injury has usually, but not always, been reversible following discontinuation of the ketoconazole. This azole is generally not used in the treatment of onychomycosis, with its main application being diseases requiring short-course therapies, for example, in pityriasis versicolor. Ketoconazole may also be considered for the treatment of vaginal candidiasis and chronic mucocutaneous candidiasis. The usual dose for the management of dermatomycoses is 200 mg/day. At higher doses there is an increased likelihood of observing endocrine adverse effects.

16.3
Topical Antifungal Agents for the Treatment of Onychomycosis

In the 1980s and 1990s, the topical antimycotic agents such as 8% ciclopirox lacquer, 5% amorolfine lacquer, and 28% tioconazole have been developed, taking advantage of new galenical preparations and transungual delivery systems [5–7].

The topical antifungal agents have been found to be safe and well tolerated, with adverse effects being confined to the site of application. The adverse effects include pruritus, burning, erythema, vesicles, stinging around the nail bed, pain and paronychia. A contact dermatitis may occur in some instances. Chromonychia following the daily use (rather than the prescribed frequency of once weekly) of amorolfine 5% lacquer has been reported [8]. There have been no reports of adverse systemic reactions with amorolfine [9] and ciclopirox olamine [Kraemer K, (May 1996) personal communication]. Thus, there are no monitoring requirements with the topical antifungal agents.

16.4
Use of Surgery Techniques and Chemical Avulsion in the Management of Onychomycosis

In selected instances, nail avulsion can be a useful adjunct to topical or oral therapies for onychomycosis. The nail avulsion can be carried out surgically [10–12] or non-surgically [13–22]. Compared with surgical avulsion, the non-surgical approach may be less expensive, cause less pain, carry a reduced risk of hemorrhage or infection, and be used in patients receiving anticoagulants [13]. The disadvantages of the non-surgical approach include the fact that it is time-consuming and the patient may inadvertently apply outdated urea preparations [13]. The earlier formulations contained urea and salicylic acid, with the addition of topical antifungal agents in the subsequent preparations. These antimycotics have included 1% bifonazole and 40% urea [17–19] as well as 2% tolnaftate ointment and 20% urea [20]. Chemical avulsion may be of benefit in onychomycosis caused by dermatophytes, yeasts [21] and other non-dermatophytes [22]. Another form of surgical management of onychomycosis is the use of a laser [23–27]. Reducing the volume of infected nail by cutting it back, curetting, and other debridement techniques may also enhance the therapeutic response.

16.5
The New Generation of Oral Antifungal Agents for the Treatment of Onychomycosis

With oral antifungal agents, systemic effects may be observed, sometimes of a serious enough nature to necessitate discontinuation of therapy. The salient adverse-effects profile of itraconazole, terbinafine, and fluconazole will now be considered [5].

16.5.1
Itraconazole

Itraconazole was the first of the new generation of antifungals to be approved in the United States for the management of onychomycosis. This agent has been prescribed to approximately 40 million patients worldwide over the last 15 years for both dermatologic and systemic conditions. In the 4 years following its approval for the treatment of toenail onychomycosis, itraconazole has been used in the United States for over 34 million patient days. This triazole has a favorable adverse-effects profile. In patients receiving itraconazole pulse therapy (200 mg twice daily for 1 week a month for 2–3 months) for the management of onychomycosis, adverse events have been reported in 11% of patients [28]. The corresponding figures with continuous therapy (200 mg/day for 3 months) and placebo are 19.6% and 15.2%, respectively [28]. Adverse events include gastrointestinal disorders (e.g. nausea, vomiting, diarrhea, abdominal pain), cutaneous eruption, pruritus, headache, malaise, vertigo, myalgia, hypertension, orthostatic hypotension, and vasculitis. Abnormal liver function tests may occur in 0.7–4% of patients receiving itraconazole therapy for onychomycosis.

The coadministration of itraconazole with astemizole, terfenadine, and cisapride, simvastatin and lovastatin is contraindicated since the metabolism of these drugs may be inhibited. Elevated levels of the first three drugs can cause cardiac adverse events. Furthermore, the coadministration of midazolam and triazolam with itraconazole are contraindicated since there may be a potentiation and prolongation of the hypnotic and sedative effects of the first two drugs. Coadministration of the following drugs with itraconazole may result in elevated levels of these drugs or an enhancement of their activity: cyclosporine, tacrolimus, digoxin, coumarin-like drugs, and oral hypoglycemics. The basis of some of the drug interactions is that itraconazole inhibits the hepatic cytochrome P450 3A4 system, which is responsible for their metabolism. Interactions may also occur between itraconazole and quinidine, vincristine, and dihydropyridine calcium channel blockers. Reduced plasma concentrations of itraconazole may occur when coadministered with the following drugs that induce hepatic cytochrome P450 enzymes: phenytoin, rifampin, and carbamazepine. Concomitant administration of itraconazole and phenytoin may also alter the metabolism of the latter; therefore, in such a context phenytoin levels should be monitored. The bioavailability of itraconazole is reduced if it is coadministered with H_2-antagonists or antacids.

With pulse therapy, there are no monitoring guidelines. In the United States, periodic liver function tests are recommended for all patients receiving continuous itraconazole for a duration exceeding 1 month, in patients with preexisting hepatic dysfunction, and in any patient who develops symptoms or signs suggestive of hepatic dysfunction.

16.5.2
Terbinafine

Terbinafine is an allylamine antifungal agent that has been used worldwide in approximately 7.5 million patients [5, 29]. It was discovered in the late 1970s and became available in the United Kingdom in 1991 and in Canada in 1993. It was approved in the United States in May 1996 for the treatment of onychomycosis. The frequency of adverse events with terbinafine has been reported to be 10.4% [30]. In another series, the corresponding figures for terbinafine and placebo were 46.7% and 29.2%, respectively [31]. Adverse events include gastrointestinal symptoms (e.g., diarrhea, dyspepsia, nausea, and abdominal pain), cutaneous eruption, pruritus, headache, and change in the ability to concentrate. Liver enzyme abnormalities may occur in 0.1–1.9% of patients and taste disturbances in 0.125% of subjects.

Terbinafine minimally activates cytochrome P450; therefore, it has a low potential for interacting with drugs metabolized through this pathway. The following drug interactions have been reported with terbinafine: rifampin (a cytochrome P450 inducer) increases terbinafine clearance by 100%, cimetidine (a cytochrome P450 inhibitor) decreases terbinafine clearance by 33%, and terfenadine decreases terbinafine clearance by 16%. Terbinafine decreases the clearance of intravenously administered caffeine by 19% and increases the clearance of cyclosporine by 15%. In normal subjects, terbinafine may not affect the clearance of antipyrine or digoxin.

In the United States, it is recommended that hepatic enzymes should be performed in patients receiving terbinafine for longer than 6 weeks [31]. Also, in patients with known or suspected immunodeficiency, physicians should consider monitoring the complete blood count when terbinafine therapy is given for periods exceeding 6 weeks [31].

16.5.3
Fluconazole

Fluconazole is a synthetic bis-triazole antifungal agent which is active against dermatophytes and *Candida* species. In North America, fluconazole is not approved for the treatment of onychomycosis. In systemic mycoses, 16% of 4048 patients experienced adverse effects in clinical trials lasting 7 days or longer [32]. The more frequently observed adverse events were gastrointestinal disturbances (nausea, vomiting, abdominal pain, diarrhea), cutaneous eruption, and headache. Approximately 5.1% of patients treated for superficial infection may have abnormal results from one or more liver function tests [33]. In patients receiving placebo therapy or applying clotrimazole, 3.7% of patients may be expected to have abnormal liver function tests [33]. Coadministration of cisapride is contraindicated with fluconazole.

Coadministration of the following drugs with fluconazole may result in an increase in the level of the drug or an enhancement of its activity: cyclosporine, especially with doses of fluconazole exceeding 100 mg/day; warfarin; sulfonylurea-oral hypoglycemics; phenytoin; and theophylline. When hydrochlorothiazide is administered concomitantly with fluconazole, there is an increase in fluconazole plasma levels, but this is felt not to be clinically significant. Coadministration of fluconazole and rifampin may result in diminished levels of the former. Cardiac dysrhythmias have occurred in patients receiving azoles in conjunction with astemizole or terfenadine. Therefore, the coadministration of these antihistamines with fluconazole should be carefully monitored.

There are no monitoring guidelines concerning the use of fluconazole for the treatment of onychomycosis.

16.6 Conclusions

The adverse effects reported with the topical antifungal agents are localized to the sites of application, and are relatively minor compared with the spectrum of adverse events that may occur with the oral antifungal agents. Therefore, when considering the optimal drug for the treatment of onychomycosis, the risk-benefit ratio of the available antifungal agents should be carefully evaluated.

References

1. Gupta AK, Sauder DN, Shear NH (1994) Antifungal agents: an overview. Part I. J Am Acad Dermatol 30:677-698
2. Sherertz EF (1990) Are laboratory studies necessary for griseofulvin therapy? J Am Acad Dermatol 22:1103
3. Jones HE (1982) Ketoconazole. Arch Dermatol 118:217-219
4. Knight TE, Shikuma CY, Knight J (1991) Ketoconazole-induced fulminant hepatitis necessitating liver transplantation. J Am Acad Dermatol 25:398-400
5. Gupta AK, Sauder DN, Shear NH (1994) Antifungal agents: an overview. Part II. J Am Acad Dermatol 30:911-933
6. Pittrof F, Gerhards J, Erni W et al (1992) Loceryl nail lacquer - realization of a new galenical approach to onychomycosis therapy. Clin Exp Dermatol 17 [Suppl 1]:26-28
7. Baran R (1993) Amorolfine nail lacquer: a new transungual delivery system for nail mycoses. JAMA [Southeast Asia Supplement] 9:5-6
8. Rigopoulos D, Katsambas A, Antoniou C et al (1996) Discoloration of the nail plate due to the misuse of amorolfine 5% nail lacquer. Acta Derm Venereol 76:83-84
9. Reinel D (1992) Topical treatment of onychomycosis with amorolfine 5% nail lacquer: comparative efficacy and tolerability of once and twice weekly use. Dermatology 184 [Suppl 1]:21-24
10. Salasche SJ (1990) Surgery. In: Scher RK, Daniel CR III (eds) Nails: therapy, diagnosis, surgery. Saunders, Philadelphia, pp 258-280
11. Haneke E, Baran R (1994) Nail surgery and traumatic abnormalities. In: Baran R, Dawber RPR (eds) Diseases of the nails and their management, 2nd edn. Blackwell Science Publications, Oxford, pp 345-416
12. Baran R, Hay RJ (1985) Partial surgical avulsion of the nail in onychomycosis. Clin Exp Dermatol 10:413-418
13. Cohen PR, Scher RK (1994) Topical and surgical treatment of onychomycosis. J Am Acad Dermatol 31:S74-77

14. Farber EM, South DA (1994) Urea ointment in the nonsurgical avulsion of nail dystrophies. Cutis 22:689–692
15. South DA, Farber EM (1980) Urea ointment in the nonsurgical avulsion of nail dystrophies – a reappraisal. Cutis 25:609–612
16. Buselmeier TJ (1980) Combination urea and salicylic acid ointment nail avulsion in nondystrophic nails: a follow-up observation. Cutis 25:397–405
17. Hay RJ, Roberts DT, Doherty VR et al (1988) The topical treatment of onychomycosis using a new combined urea/imidazole preparation. Clin Exp Dermatol 13:164–167
18. Bonifaz A, Guzman A, Garcia C et al (1995) Efficacy and safety of bifonazole urea in the two-phase treatment of onychomycosis. Int J Dermatol 34:500–501
19. Fritsch H (1992) Ultrastructural changes in onychomycosis during the treatment with bifonazole/urea ointment. Dermatology 185:32–36
20. Ishii M, Hamada T, Asai Y (1983) Treatment of onychomycosis by ODT therapy with 20% urea ointment and 2% tolnaftate ointment. Dermatologica 167:273–279
21. White MI, Clayton YM (1982) The treatment of fungus and yeast infections of nails by the method of chemical removal. Clin Exp Dermatol 7:273–276
22. Rollman O, Johansson S (1987) Hendersonula toruloidea infection: successful response of onychomycosis to nail avulsion and topical ciclopiroxolamine. Acta Derm Venereol 67:506–510
23. Leshin B, Whitaker DC (1988) Carbon dioxide laser matricectomy. J Dermatol Surg Oncol 14:608–611
24. Scher RK (1981) Surgical avulsion of nail plates by a proximal to distal technique. J Dermatol Surg Oncol 7:296–297
25. Rothermel E, Apfelberg DB (1987) Carbon dioxide laser use for certain diseases of the toenails. Clin Podiatr Med Surg 4:809–821
26. Geronemus RG (1992) Laser surgery of the nail unit. J Dermatol Surg Oncol 18:735–743
27. Apfelberg DB, Rothermel E, Eidtfeldt A et al (1984) Preliminary report on use of carbon dioxide laser in podiatry. J Am Podiatr Med Assoc 74:509–513
28. Gupta AK, De Doncker P, Scher RK et al (1997) Itraconazole for the treatment of onychomycosis: an overview. Dermatologic Clinics 15:121–135
29. Shear NH, Gupta AK (1995) Terbinafine for the treatment of pedal onychomycosis: a foot closer to the promised land of cured nails? Arch Dermatol 131:937–942
30. Sandoz Inc. (1995) Terbinafine product monograph. Sandoz Inc., Dorval, Québec
31. Sandoz Inc. (1996) Terbinafine product monograph. Sandoz Inc., New Jersey, USA
32. Pfizer Inc. (1994) Fluconazole product monograph. Pfizer Inc., Kirkland, Québec
33. Hay RJ (1993) Risk/benefit ratio of modern antifungal therapy: focus on hepatic reactions. J Am Acad Dermatol 29:S50–S54

CHAPTER 17

Differential Diagnosis of Onychomycosis and Rationale for a Step-Therapy in Treating Nail Fungal Infection

R. Baran

17.1 Introduction

Onychomycosis is so frequently encountered in daily practice that any nail dystrophy, especially in isolation, may lead clinically to a wrong diagnosis. For example:
- Distal lateral subungual onychomycosis with subungual hyperkeratosis can be mimicked by psoriasis, Reiter's syndrome, pityriasis rubra pilaris, Norwegian scabies, Darier's disease, lichen planus, chronic dermatitis, erythroderma, pachyonychia congenita, and acrokeratosis paraneoplastica.
- Distal lateral subungual onychomycosis with onycholysis may be simulated by repeated microtrauma to the great toenail or by other rarer causes such as subungual tumors.
- Proximal subungual onychomycosis can masquerade as trivial leuconychia, leuconychic psoriasis, or neurological disorder (sympathetic reflex, C4 spinal cord injury, etc.).
- Proximal subungual onychomycosis with paronychia, a condition usually caused by *Candida* infection, may be impossible to differentiate clinically from *Fusarium* infection and many other dermatological conditions.
- Onychomycotic melanonychia, hematoma, subungual tumors, longitudinal melanonychia, and even malignant melanoma should be ruled out.

Since differential diagnosis is discussed here only on clinical grounds according to the major features observed in the nail apparatus, the diagnosis of onychomycosis must be confirmed in the laboratory. In the nail conditions mentioned above, neither hyphae nor spores are found in the cornified cells of the nail bed or in the lowest portion of the nail plate. However, dual pathologies do occur and psoriatic nails, particularly toenails, may be associated with commensal fungi as colonization caused by *Candida* or, more rarely, a dermatophyte.

The management of onychomycosis entails systemic antifungal drug treatment, local antifungals, or avulsion, surgical (partial) or chemical.

17.2
Oral Antifungal Agents

With the new systemic antifungal drugs, which are still under investigation in some countries, the rationale for treating onychomycosis has changed. The newer triazoles, fluconazole and itraconazole and the oral allylamine, terbinafine, differ from the traditional antifungal drugs because of rapid penetration into the nail via the nail bed and/or their binding to matrix tissue, allowing drug retention in the nail plate after discontinuation of therapy. This produces continuous improvement, which allows short-duration treatment and even intermittent therapy.

17.2.1
Itraconazole

Itraconazole [1, 2] has the broadest in vitro spectrum of the oral antifungal drugs. It is effective against dermatophytes, *Candida*, and some nondermatophyte molds. Owing to an unusual pharmacokinetic profile, with a high affinity to nail keratin [3], the recommended schedule is 200 mg b.i.d. daily, for 1 week per month [4] in an à-la-carte treatment regimen lasting 1–2 months for fingernail infections and 3–4 months for toenails. Although the nail will not be normal when therapy is discontinued, improvement continues, sometimes at a slower rate than during the treatment period, when an increase in linear nail growth may be observed [5].

17.2.2
Fluconazole

Fluconazole [1, 2], which is active against *Candida* and other yeasts, as well as dermatophytes, has been used widely in HIV-infected patients. It was thought that, as with griseofulvin and ketoconazole, long-term therapy would usually require consistently repeated doses. This opinion has to be revised [6], and 150 mg administered once a week may be a useful intermittent regimen [7] in patients taking multiple medications.

17.2.3
Terbinafine

Terbinafine [1, 2, 8] is the only in vitro fungicidal oral antifungal with activity against the dermatophytes, some species of *Candida*, and even some molds. It is detectable in the nail plate in 1–3 weeks and persists for up to 4 months after therapy is discontinued. A 12-week course of 250 mg once a day is effective in toenail infections [9], while 6 weeks of therapy are sufficient for fingernail disease. As with itraconazole, the nail will not be clinically normal when the drug is discontinued, but because terbinafine is retained in its keratin, the nail plate grows out healthy.

Potent systemic therapy may, however, be limited by severe adverse reactions. In addition, some patients are unwilling or unable to take oral drugs. Topical application directly onto the nail plate would thus be an attractive alternative.

17.3
Topical Antifungal Agents

In the past topical therapy has not been very successful in the treatment of onychomycosis. As an explanation for this there are several reasons.

The nail plate is a special obstacle which prevents topically applied drug substances to reach the site of infection in the nail bed. The nail plate is derived from an invagination, the proximal nail groove, which has a roof, the proximal nail fold and a floor, the nail matrix. The nail plate emerges from beneath the proximal nail fold which adheres closely to the dorsum of the nail for a short distance and forms a gradually desquamating tissue, the cuticle which seals the proximal nail groove. The proximal nail fold is contiguous with the similarly structured lateral nail fold on each side.

The nail plate protects the half-moon shaped white lunula which represents the distal portion of the matrix and the pink nail bed. Distally, adjacent to the nail bed, the hyponychium, an extension of the epidermis under the nail plate, marks the point at which the nail separates from the underlying tissue.

The ventral layer of the nail plate adheres firmly to the nail bed, whereas adherence to the nail matrix is poor.

Due to the fact that the lateral edges of the nail plate sit somewhat loosely in the lateral nail grooves even the new systemic drugs that penetrate the nail keratin in a few days via the nail bed give a poor response in lateral nail disease for reasons explained by the anatomy of the nail organ (10–11).

Unfortunately, in the past topical formulations were not specifically adapted to the nail organ, which is an obstacle to successful treatment of onychomycosis:
1. Conventional formulations do not guarantee a sufficient liberation of the antifungal agent, which is the main prerequisite for penetration of the nail barrier.
2. They are not adapted to the usual treatment duration required for the regrowth of a healthy nail because they do not remain in contact with the site of application for a long period of time.

To ensure successful topical therapy, therefore, the drug used has to meet the following requirements:
- Highly effective antifungal agent
- Suitable system providing high liberation of the drug from the vehicle
- Complete and rapid penetration of the nail plate

- Fungicidal drug concentration at the site of the infection
- Ease and convenience of application.

Transungual penetration by the appropriate drug is the prerequisite for effective topical therapy. Penetration of the nail plate by the drug is dependent on three factors (12):
  I. The physicochemical properties of the nail
  II. The physicochemical properties of the compound
  III. The vehicle containing the active agent

I. Physicochemical properties of the Nail
- The entire nail structure is made of hard keratin and the outermost dorsal layer is especially dense (13). The hardness of the nail plate depends on the junctions between the cells and their architectural arrangement. Moreover, the multiplicity of the lateral bonds between keratin fibers (disulfide bridges, hydrogen bonds, acid-base bonds, electrostatic bonds) accounts also for the high resistance of nail keratin to penetration by an agent.
- The nail plate is relatively chemically inert, given that it is a cornified epithelial structure. In terms of its composition the nail plate is more like hair than stratum corneum (13). Proteins are its major component. The nail plate contains cholesterol as the main lipid acting as a plasticizer.
- In fact, the main nail plasticizer is water. The ideal proportion of water in nail tissue is 18% and is directly related to ambient relative humidity. The permeability of nail by water is some thousandfold greater than that of the stratum corneum.

The hydrophilic nature of the nail means that it is the hydrophilic pathway rather than the lipophilic which is responsible for rapid penetration by water and highly water-soluble compounds such as urea and methanol (13).

II. The Properties of the Drug
The compound chosen should be an appropriate keratinophilic drug. Molecular weight and size as well as the lipophilic/hydrophilic profile have to be taken into account. Many polar and non-polar substances with widely differing molecular weight (30 to 665) are able to penetrate the nail (12). The use of transungual penetration promoter such as DMSO is equivocal. Stüttgen (14) claims that DMSO enhances permeation inside the deeper keratin layers. On the other hand, Walters (13) found no indication that DMSO can accelerate the penetrability of the nail plate. (Solvents which tend to promote penetration of the skin horny layer show little promise as accelerants of nail plate penetrability.) Moreover, DMSO was even found to retard penetration by methanol and hexanol, while isopropyl alcohol reduces the penetration rate only of hexanol through the nail plate. Nevertheless, there is evidence that sodium lauryl sulfate, sodium sulfide and sodium thioglycolate are penetration enhancers (13).

III. The Vehicle containing the active Agent
We know that the method of delivery in use on skin is inappropriate for releasing active agents onto the nail, despite the addition of penetration enhancers [10, 11]. This explains attempts to improve the conventional topical treatments:

1. Modifications of the vehicle pH have been used, as in the case of miconazole, where a high concentration of the active agent is achieved by decreasing the formulation pH, thereby increasing drug solubility in the vehicle for maximal diffusion.
2. New simple formulations such as Faergeman's solution (lactic acid, urea, propylene glycol) or 28% tioconazole or 40% urea have been used. The two former solutions have produced only moderate results, and urea paste acts principally on the pathological nail plate-nail bed attachment. Nonsurgical avulsion with a urea-based preparation such as bifonazole-urea eradicates the pathogens. However, this antifungal chemotherapeutic keratinolysis has some drawbacks: it is cumbersome if several nails are involved, inefficient when the nail is affected beneath the proximal nail fold, and fungi may still be present under the margin of the remaining normal nail keratin adherent to the nail bed.
3. A real step forward has been achieved with the development of a new vehicle in the form of a cosmetic nail lacquer, the film-forming polymer reducing transungual water loss. Because of this formulation, the nail lacquer maintains the active agent in the polymer film reservoir on the nail surface from which the chemical diffuses evenly through the nail keratin to reach the nail bed [12, 16-18]. After evaporation of the solvent in the nail lacquer, the concentration of the diffusion molecule in the film increases, which in turn enhances penetration and diffusion.

Release and rate of diffusion can be optimized by selecting the components of the lacquer formulation, which helps to modulate the release of the drug into the nail plate and maintains the antifungal at a high level. Two antifungal drugs, amorolfine [18] and ciclopirox [19] are currently used in this type of formulation as transungual antifungal delivery systems.

Taking into account fungal involvement of the lunula portion, the lateral edge of the nail, and the subungual area (which may lead to large onycholysis), a rationale for a step-therapy approach in treating onychomycosis can be proposed. The first-line therapy for fungal involvement of the distal two-thirds of the nail plate is topical monotherapy with the nail lacquers, which acts as a transungual drug delivery system. Such a treatment at the beginning of the mycotic process of distal subungual onychomycosis solves the problem of retaining the active agent in contact with the substrate for a long enough time to produce the desired antifungal action. This therapy is, however, inappropriate in more severe cases presenting with lunula involvement and lateral nail disease [11] or onycholysis, where the nail plate is no longer in contact with the subungual tissue (thereby interrupting the transport process of the drug from the nail into the nail bed). This drawback is also encountered with the new systemic antifungal drugs that penetrate the nail via the nail bed. Nevertheless, they still penetrate the nail keratin through the matrix; however, the clinical and mycological response may be diminished. Consequently, our therapeutic strategy leads, now, to a step-therapy approach, involving either antifungal nail lacquer alone in mild cases, or combined therapy of antifungal nail lacquers with the new systemic drugs. This must sometimes be supplemented by chemical avulsion to eliminate onycholysis, lateral nail disease, and "walled off" infection [20] to obtain the best therapeutic results in the shortest time. It also minimizes the risk of adverse effects of the systemic drugs and lowers the cost of treatment.

Such a combination therapy is beneficial since it eradicates fungal foci in the nail plate with the topical treatment as well as in the nail bed with the systemic antifungals; the latter also permit oral therapy of tinea pedis, which often precedes onychomycosis. Additionally, the new systemic antimycotic agents and transungual drug delivery systems may utilize compounds that act on different potential targets for antifungal chemotherapy. On the one hand, the new systemic drugs inhibit the membrane sterol biosynthesis, which affects the cytoplasmic membrane, and on the other hand, ciclopirox, for example, acts as a metabolic inhibitor, mainly on the respiratory chain of the fungal cell, thus making a key step towards the inaccessible goal of a 100% success rate. Another goal of great importance is the identification of those patients who require this approach.

Finally, long-term intermittent therapy should prevent recurrence of tinea pedis and limit the possibility of reinfection. Periodic use of transungual drug delivery systems, which are retained in nail keratin after discontinuation of therapy, appears to be a logical and safe method for preventing recurrences.

References

1. Gupta AK, Sauder DN, Shear NH (1994) Antifungal agents. Part II. J Am Acad Dermatol 30:911–933
2. Elewski BE (1994) Onychomycosis. Fitzpatrick's J Clin Dermatol
3. Matthieu L, De Doncker P, Cauwenbergh G et al (1991) Itraconazole penetrates the nail via the nail matrix and the nail bed: an investigation in onychomycosis. Clin Exp Dermatol 16:374–376
4. Roseew D, De Doncker P (1993) New approaches to the treatment of onychomycosis. J Am Acad Dermatol 29:545–550
5. De Doncker P, Pierard G (1994) Acquired nail beading in patients on itraconazole: an indicator of faster nail growth? Clin Exp Dermatol 19:404–406
6. Faergemann J, Laufen H (1996) Levels of fluconazole in normal and diseased nails during and after treatment of onychomycoses in toenails with fluconazole 150 mg once weekly. Acta Derm Venereol 76:219–221
7. Suchil P, Montero-Gei F, Robles M et al (1992) Once-weekly oral doses of fluconazole 150 mg in the treatment of tinea corporis/cruris and cutaneous candidiasis. Clin Exp Dermatol 17:397–401
8. Shear NH, Gupta AK (1995) Terbinafine for the treatment of pedal onychomycosis. A foot closer to the promised land of cured nails. Arch Dermatol 131:937–942
9. Goodfield MJ (1992) Short-duration therapy with terbinafine for dermatophyte onychomycosis. A multicenter trial. Br J Dermatol 126:33–35
10. Baran R (1994) Cosmetology of normal nails. In: Cosmetic Dermatology, Baran R. & Maibach H. (Eds.). Martin Dunitz, London, chap 6–7, pp 157–167.
11. Baran R & de Doncker P (1996) Lateral edge nail involvement indicates poor prognosis for treating onychomycosis with the new systemic antifungals. In: Acta Derm Venereol, 76, pp 82–83
12. Marty JP (1995) Amorolfine nail lacquer: a novel formulation. In: JEADV, 4:suppl 1, pp 17–21
13. Walters KA, Flynn GL (1983) Permeability characteristics of the human nail plate. Int J Cosmet Sci 5:231–246
14. Stüttgen G, Bauer E (1982) Bioavailability, skin- and nailpenetration of topically applied antimycotics. Mykosen 25:74–80

15. Cesquin-Roques CG, Hänel H, Pruja-Bougaret SM, Vandermander J, Michel G (1991) Ciclopirox nail lacquer 8%. In vivo penetration into and through nails and in vitro effect on pig skin. Skin Pharmacol 4:89–94
16. Polak A (1993) Kinetics of amorolfin in human nails. Mycoses 36:101–103
17. Baran R (1993) Amorolfine nail lacquer. A new transungual delivery system for nail mycoses. JAMA Southeast Asia 9 [Suppl 4]:5–6
18. Zaug M (1995) Amorolfine nail lacquer: clinical experience in onychomycosis. JEADV 4 [Suppl 1]:S23–S30
19. Meisel CW, Nietsch P (1992) Ein neues Therapiekonzept bei Onychomykosen. Dtsch Dermatol 7:1038–1053
20. Robert DT (1996) What is the relationship between therapeutic regimens, treatment duration and treatment failure in onychomycosis. Sandoz satellite symposium: Fifth EADV Congress. Lisbon Oct 14

Printing and Binding: Druckhaus Beltz, Hemsbach